# Fine Needle Aspiration
## of Palpable Masses

# Fine Needle Aspiration of Palpable Masses

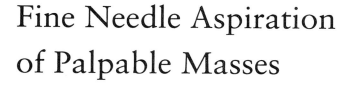
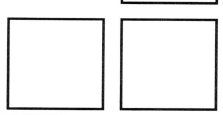

## MICHAEL W. STANLEY, M.D.

*Associate Professor of Pathology*
*Director of Cytopathology*
*Department of Pathology*
*The College of Medicine*

and

*Medical Director*
*Department of Cytotechnology*
*College of Health Related Professions*
*University of Arkansas for Medical Sciences*
*Little Rock, Arkansas*

## TORSTEN LÖWHAGEN, M.D., F.I.A.C.

*Associate Head*
*Division of Clinical Cytology*
*Department of Pathology*
*Karolinska Hospital*
*Stockholm, Sweden*

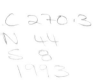
## Butterworth–Heinemann

Boston   London   Oxford   Singapore   Sydney   Toronto   Wellington

Every effort has been made to ensure that the drug dosage schedules within this text are accurate
and conform to standards accepted at time of publication. However, as treatment recommendations vary in the light of continuing research and clinical experience, the reader is advised to
verify drug dosage schedules herein with information found on product information sheets. This
is especially true in cases of new or infrequently used drugs.

Recognizing the importance of preserving what has been written, it is the policy of Butterworth–
Heinemann to have the books it publishes printed on acid-free paper, and we exert our best
efforts to that end.

**Library of Congress Cataloging-in-Publication Data**
Stanley, Michael W.
    Fine needle aspiration of palpable masses / Michael W. Stanley,
  Torsten Löwhagen.
       p.    cm.
    Includes bibliographical references and index.
    ISBN 0-7506-9455-6 (case : alk. paper)
    1. Biopsy, Needle.  2. Tumors—Cytodiagnosis.    I. Löwhagen,
  Torsten.    II. Title.
    [DNLM: 1. Biopsy, Needle—methods.    WB 379 S788f]
  RC270.3.N44S8      1993
  616.07'58—dc20
  DNLM/DLC                  92-49527

**British Library Cataloguing-in-Publication Data**
A catalogue record for this book is available from the British Library.

Butterworth–Heinemann
80 Montvale Avenue
Stoneham, MA 02180

10  9  8  7  6  5  4  3  2  1

Printed in the United States of America

*To Michelle and Anna-Stina: The Why That Informs How*

# Contents

# *Preface*

FNA is a direct, first-line approach to the evaluation of palpable masses. The logical first step of quickly, painlessly, and inexpensively obtaining material for a tissue diagnosis is frequently delayed while indirect or tangential radiographic and laboratory investigations are pursued. These time-consuming, expensive, and sometimes anxiety-provoking tests often seem unnecessary when the FNA results are finally available.

One must ask why a valuable clinical method that was developed in America was first used extensively in Sweden. Its initial applications were by Nils Söderstrom and Sixten Franzen. Franzen was a clinical hematologist–oncologist who was subsequently joined by the pathologist, Joseph Zajicek. Thus, the method that was implemented by clinicians and organized by a pathologist became a clinical-oncology unit staffed by diagnostic pathologists who evolved into clinician–pathologist hybrids. The method rapidly became indispensable to the practice of clinical oncology; the cytology clinic at the Karolinska Hospital is housed in the oncology facility at the insistence of the Department of Medical Oncology. In this model, clinician support of pathologist involvement in clinical medicine is essential.

The great challenge today is to train cytopathologists to bring the benefits of this discipline to the patients who could benefit from it. We hope that this book will contribute to this important effort. We must temper our wish for its success with a word of caution. Words and pictures will never suffice to transmit manual and intellectual diagnostic skills. Person-to-person exchange in teaching and learning must ultimately form the basis for expanding the new discipline of clinical cytopathology. We hope that this book will provide focus, organization, and objectives; it can never replace the master–apprentice relationship on which teaching in medicine is ultimately based.

# Acknowledgments

We gratefully acknowledge the advice, encouragement, and support of our friends and colleagues in the clinical, cytology, and pathology departments at our institutions. Without this support, this book would never have been completed. As always, chief among them is Chuck. We are also deeply grateful to Ms. Terry Joncas for her continuous typing and retyping of the manuscript. Her cheerfulness belies the great burden we added to her already endless list of tasks.

Two individuals have kindly shared high-quality photographs of their important clinical material. We are indebted to Dr. John Knoedler (Figures 2.2, 3.10, and 3.11) and to Dr. Charles A. Horwitz (Figures 1.2, 1.42, 1.52, 2.19, and 2.26). Ms. Ida Phillips prepared the line drawings in Figures 1.14, 2.1, 2.7 through 2.10, 2.12, 2.24, and 2.25. Her skill is much admired and appreciated. We gratefully acknowledge permission of the publishers to reprint Figures 1.5, 1.11 through 1.14, and 1.27 from our previous contribution to *The Oxford Textbook of Pathology*. Mr. Brian Coria prepared many of the photographs of slides, smears, and equipment. Mr. Michael Morris of the University of Arkansas Graphics Center assisted with many aspects of black-and-white photography. The cytologic material used for illustrative purposes was stained and cataloged by Ms. Pauline Fruetel.

All physicians involved in clinical FNA owe a great debt to those who developed it so extensively. Chief among these are Dr. Sixten Franzen and Dr. Joseph Linsk, as made clear in their book *Fine Needle Aspiration for the Clinician* (J.B. Lippincott Co., Philadelphia, 1986). Dr. Joseph Zajicek did much to solidify the relationship between histopathology and aspiration cytopathology.

# Introduction

Considering the rapid proliferation of articles, symposia, tutorials, and books dedicated to diagnosis of mass lesions by fine-needle aspiration cytology, those proposing to burden the physician and the cytotechnologist with yet another volume of techniques, tips, and personal observations should be prepared to present good reasons why their book is a needed addition. This is especially so because many seem to regard this method as so simple that its technical aspects hardly need be described at all, let alone discussed at length. If this were so, we would not receive on a daily basis uninterpretable smears obtained with relatively large needles through multiple punctures of unhappy patients.

When reduced to its simplest terms, FNA consists of (1) using a needle and a syringe to remove material from a mass, (2) smearing it on a glass slide, (3) applying a routine stain, and (4) looking at it with a clinical microscope. The lofty goal of this simple process is no less than rapid, accurate, and nearly painless diagnosis of the vast majority of mass lesions. Achieving this goal by such simple means demands that each step in the process be optimized. Some tumors can be diagnosed by almost any clinical technique, coupled with any degree of laboratory expertise, but achieving the goal just outlined is much more difficult. It is to this end that we offer a compendium of clinical and laboratory techniques that we have found useful in our daily work. Many of these have been developed by the group at the Karolinska Hospital and passed willingly to student guests from around the world. It is in this way that the junior (MWS) author was taught by the senior author.

Our aim, then, is not to justify FNA as a clinical technique, but rather to suggest some methods that have been shown to work exceedingly well. Our suggestions are directed to those who already recognize the value of FNA in patient care. From the outset, we acknowledge that nothing we describe can be accomplished by our methods alone. Other approaches have their adherents, many of whom practice brilliantly.

Several aspects of this practice, although very important, do not receive detailed descriptions here. These include standard techniques common to most cytopathology laboratories that have some utility in FNA, such as recipes for routine stains and centrifugation techniques. Methods for special studies such as cell-surface-marker analysis, electron microscopy, and immunocytochemistry for tumor typing are mentioned briefly, but the details of their execution are left to the many excellent references in these specialized fields.

Because this is a methods book written for those already convinced that FNA is a valuable clinical tool, we do not discuss such issues as false-positive and false-negative rates. Many authors have already addressed the quantitative aspects of these topics in detail, and indeed, they form a critical part of the historical development of this diagnostic method. Those wishing to review the accuracy rates for FNA of various sites should consult the standard textbooks or should review historical aspects of the method. False-positive diagnoses almost always arise from problems in microscopic interpretation and are thus beyond the scope of this book. In a sense, this whole treatise is about minimizing false negatives by using proper clinical and laboratory techniques.

Complications of FNA are exceedingly rare, and some are mentioned in Chapter 2. This is done in the context of specific body sites in which a given complication might seem likely to occur. Those discussions are brief and cite a small number of important references.

Photomicrographs are shown mostly as a way of illustrating technical points or of demonstrating the nature of good-quality specimens. They underscore our discussions of specimen cellularity, cell preservation, smear preparation, and staining quality. We also hope that this glimpse through the microscope will enable clinicians to appreciate the nature of cytologic diagnoses and improve communication with the laboratory about problem cases. No attempt has been made to prepare an atlas of cytopathology.

The format of this book is as follows: Chapter 1 describes the basic techniques of needle aspiration. Methods for preparing the material obtained for micros-copy are illustrated, as are routine stains and rapid stains. A comparison of the two most commonly used stains is offered. Chapter 2 discusses clinical tech-niques and results reporting. These include ways of answering commonly asked questions from patients and their physicians. Chapter 3 uses a series of case studies to illustrate the power of diagnosis by aspiration of palpable masses with thin needles. These cases are also used to illustrate technical points made in the first two chapters, and to indicate additional aspects of specimen preparation.

Medicolegal issues are briefly discussed when we offer some reflections on benign breast masses. It is in this setting that the failure to diagnose cancer on a timely basis seems most likely. The section on results reporting also considers medicolegal issues and the methods of documentation needed to minimize risk.

The method that we describe has been known by several designations. We have chosen *fine-needle aspiration* (FNA); it is at once descriptive and accurate. We have carefully avoided use of the word *biopsy* because for many clinicians this connotes removal of solid tissue by surgical means (the meaning of the Greek root words not withstanding). We agree with Trott that "for purposes of communication with clinicians a distinction is needed" between aspiration with thin needles and "the procedure of needle biopsy by which a core of tissue is removed for embedding in paraffin wax and sectioning."[1] Confining the term *biopsy* to histopathology and using *aspirate* to describe material obtained by FNA was encouraged by the editors of one cytopathology journal in 1990.[2]

[1]Trott DA: Needle aspiration terminology. Acta Cytol 1983; 27:83.
[2]Coleman DV, Trott PA: Editorial. Fine needle aspiration. Cytopathol 1990;1:57–58.

# Equipment, Basic Techniques, and Staining Procedures

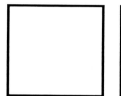

**1**

It would be difficult to think of a contemporary medical procedure that is less high tech than fine-needle aspiration (FNA). Its initial clinical application antedated by decades the development of many modern diagnostic devices.[1] At its simplest, only a needle without a syringe is required because, in some cases, capillary action will suffice to admit cells to the needle. The use of a syringe adds negative pressure to the needle tip and extends the range of lesions that can be successfully sampled using this technique.

Although FNA has always been a simple procedure, several technical improvements have occurred since its initial description. Modern needles are sterile, disposable, very sharp, and available in a wide range of diameters and lengths. The syringe holder that is described subsequently in this chapter allows the operator to have one hand completely free during the FNA procedure. This permits stabilization of target lesions, leading to accurate puncture of even very small masses. The needle guide invented by Dr. Sixten Franzen at Sweden's Karolinska Hospital permits accurate, atraumatic aspiration of palpable masses in the prostate, as well as perirectal or perivaginal masses.[2]

A successful marriage of low tech and high tech occurs when modern radiographic techniques are used to guide a long thin needle to a deep-seated, nonpalpable mass lesion. Long, flexible needles, with either metal or plastic tips, have been developed for use during endoscopy. These needles can be passed through the biopsy channel of either a gastrointestinal endoscope or a bronchoscope to sample pulmonary, mediastinal, or abdominal masses.[3]

Despite the use of radiologic or endoscopic techniques to extend the range of masses to which FNA can be applied, the basic technique remains quite simple. The same simplicity that makes FNA safe, rapid, inexpensive, and accurate can also be its most severe problem. This maneuver, though very powerful, is technically much less difficult to perform than many other common procedures, such as bone-marrow biopsy, central-venous line placement, or tracheal intubation.

We have repeatedly observed that with this assessment firmly in mind, some who are new to FNA accord its various components little attention, thereby mistaking the simple for the trivial. The wonder is that such practitioners occasionally produce diagnostically useful material. More often, however, the results of carelessly performed FNA are unsatisfactory for diagnosis. Contributing to this is the fact that those who are untutored in the procedure are often similarly unaware of reasonable methods for preparation of any material obtained, as well as for proper fixation or air drying of smears. Thus, problems at several levels of the procedure add to rendering many examinations nearly worthless. The entire process is a chain of events only as strong as its weakest link. Instruction in the basic techniques of aspiration, slide preparation, and specimen fixation or drying can greatly improve the quality of diagnostic results. Only then can the potential of FNA for accurate, high-yield diagnosis be achieved.

Whether performed in the clinic, at the bedside, in the radiology suite, or in the endoscopy laboratory, the fundamentals of FNA are constant. In this chapter, we first examine the basic equipment of FNA. Then, the technique of aspiration with small-gauge needles is discussed. We next suggest methods for preparation of aspirated material at the time of the procedure. Routine staining methods used in the cytopathology laboratory are then considered. Our goal is to describe thoroughly the actions that, when mastered following a little practice, are rapid and simple.

It is unfortunate that verbal or pictorial descriptions may cause some techniques to appear more complicated or laborious than is actually the case. The techniques we describe are simple, though they are not trivial. Having discussed and taught these ideas with many physicians new to the techniques of FNA, we are convinced that it is these small points that are responsible for success or failure in this endeavor.

We are often told that a fear of those contemplating the use of FNA is that the pathologists may be unable to interpret properly the material obtained. Certainly, interpretation of cytologic preparations is very important reflecting or echoing traditional histopathology more than actually extending it. (The recent proliferation of books on various aspects of this subject attest to this fact.) In our experience, however, more problems in FNA occur at the bedside than at the microscope. Thus, we emphasize these details of clinical aspiration.

## EQUIPMENT

### Needles

Many advantages of tumor sampling by FNA are the direct result of the small diameter of the needles typically used. These include an extremely low complication rate, excellent patient acceptance, no scars, and no need for anesthesia. Furthermore, the aspiration can be repeated, as needed, for special studies, for assessment of treatment effects, or for obtaining additional tissue for a more complete or certain diagnosis. Nordenskjold et al. describe sequential aspiration of breast-cancer patients for assessment of tumor-cell thymidine labeling and the effects of treatment on the tumor.[4] Some of their patients accepted up to 40 FNA procedures.

Figure 1.1 shows a comparison of a 2-mm tissue-core biopsy needle with the needle most often used for FNA. Most aspirations are performed with 23- to 27-gauge needles. These permit adequate sampling of a majority of masses. When a fibrous mass is encountered, or a very scant aspirate is obtained, a larger needle can be used. Rarely, we have used a 20-gauge needle for fibrous tumors. In our experience, the smallest needle that will adequately sample a given mass is to be preferred. For example, needles larger than 23-gauge, when applied to breast FNA, cause increased bleeding rather than larger specimens. For this reason, the diagnostic yield may be lower than that obtained when using smaller needles.

At the Karolinska Hospital, there has been a progression over many years toward smaller needles. Now, 27-gauge (0.4 mm) needles are often used. The samples are excellent, bleeding is minimal, and patient acceptance is very good. Furthermore, these thinner needles are passed easily through sclerotic tissue, such as that often encountered in benign breast disease.

The appropriate needle length depends on the nature of the target lesion. Using 25-gauge needles, many lymph nodes can be reached with a ⅝-inch (16 mm) length. A 1 ½-inch (3.8 cm) length can be used for many breast masses, whereas a patient with large breasts or a palpable abdominal mass may require a 2- (5 cm) or 3 ½-inch (8.8 cm) length. The 1 ½-inch, 25-gauge needle is used for the majority of our aspirations.

Figure 1.1.
*A tissue-core biopsy needle (top) is compared with a 25-gauge (0.5 mm) fine needle.*

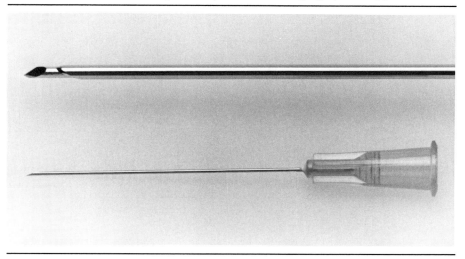

Obviously, a too-short needle will miss the lesion. In our experience, many breast masses are deeper than initial palpation may indicate. Figure 1.2 shows the results of using a needle of insufficient length. Aspiration of this breast carcinoma yielded damaged adipose tissue from the edge of the tumor and showed the cytologic pattern of fat necrosis. Had a longer needle been used, diagnostic tumor cells would probably have been obtained. As discussed in Chapters 2 and 3, the inadequacy of the aspiration specimen should probably have been realized at the time of the procedure and the aspiration repeated at once. Attention to the tissue textures as the needle was advanced and gross inspection of the aspirated material would probably have shown that the lesion had been missed and that no tissue consistent with the clinical findings had been obtained. Sizes and length of needles are summarized in Table 1.1.

We prefer needles with a plastic hub rather than a metal hub. This permits the operator to monitor the recovery of tissue or blood or other fluid as it appears in the hub. Diagnostic tissue fragments are often trapped in the needle hub. Using techniques we discuss subsequently herein, an effort should be made to recover these fragments for microscopic examination. Thus, a clear view of the needle hub and its contents is helpful. A translucent tinted hub (usually blue for 25-gauge needles) is acceptable. We have not found it necessary to allocate extra funds for purchase of special FNA needles advertised for having a clear hub.

Figure 1.2.
*Surgically resected breast mass with overlying skin shows the reason for a false negative aspiration. The needle (25-gauge, 1 ½-inch length) was too short to reach the tumor. In our experience, many breast masses are deeper than initial palpation may suggest. (Photograph courtesy of Dr. Charles A. Horwitz, Metropolitan—Mt. Sinai Hospital, Minneapolis, Minnesota.)*

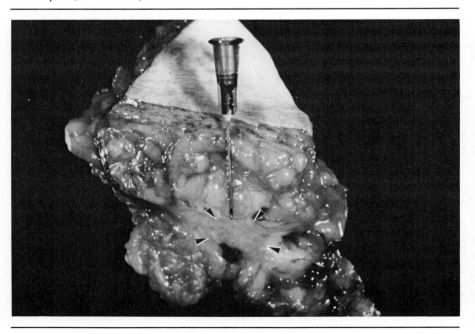

Table 1.1
*Diameter and length of needles used for fine-needle aspiration cytology*

| Gauge | Outside Diameter | Inside Diameter | Available Lengths | Lumen Cross-sectional Area (Calculated) |
|---|---|---|---|---|
| 20 | 0.89 | 0.58 | 25, 38, 76 | 0.26 mm$^2$ |
| 22 | 0.71 | 0.41 | 19, 25, 38 | 0.13 mm$^2$ |
| 23 | 0.64 | 0.33 | 6, 19, 25 | 0.09 mm$^2$ |
| 25 | 0.51 | 0.25 | 16, 25, 32, 38, 51, 88 | 0.05 mm$^2$ |
| 27 | 0.41 | 0.20 | 13, 19, 38 | 0.03 mm$^2$ |

*Note.* All measurements are in millimeters. These data were kindly provided by John Miller of Sherwood Medical Products, St. Louis, Missouri.

## Syringes

Modern sterile, disposable syringes made of clear plastic are perfect for use in FNA. Most practitioners use the 10-cc size, while some prefer the 20-cc size. We have occasionally seen use of a 3-cc syringe, and our colleagues in radiology sometimes ask for a 50- or 60-cc size. We are accustomed to using the 10-cc or 12-cc size and virtually never use other syringe types.

Some workers use glass syringes. These are expensive, require lubrication, are easily broken and must be cleaned and autoclaved between uses. Furthermore, glass syringes are not suitable for use in the syringe holder illustrated in Figure 1.3. Although we have little actual experience with glass syringes, their use seems to us a needless complication, with no obvious benefits.

Table 1.2 summarizes the luminal pressure that can be generated by evacuating syringes of various sizes. The data are calculated by using the gas law to expand the dead-space volume of the empty syringe to its maximum capacity. Using a standard Luer-tip syringe fitted with a standard-sized needle hub, the dead-space volume is approximately 0.13 cc. When the initial pressure is 760 mm Hg, expanding this volume to the maximum final volume allowed by the syringe yields the luminal pressures shown. The final column in Table 1.2 shows the difference between the ambient pressure (760 mm Hg) and the luminal

Table 1.2
*Syringe luminal pressure for different syringe volumes*

| Syringe Volume (cc) | Luminal Pressure (mm Hg) | Ambient–Syringe Pressure Difference (mm Hg) |
|---|---|---|
| 3 | 30.4 | 730 |
| 5 | 18.2 | 742 |
| 10 | 9.1 | 751 |
| 12 | 7.6 | 752 |
| 20 | 4.5 | 756 |
| 50 | 1.8 | 758 |

pressure. Clearly, in terms of the amount of suction provided, the differences among syringe sizes, as shown in the third column of the table, are trivial. Therefore, selection of a syringe size should be based on comfort, convenience, availability, and personal preference. Larger syringes do not yield larger samples.

Some practitioners make a point of preferring the type of syringe with an eccentrically located needle attachment. We have not found this to be an important issue and have used both eccentric and centered needle attachments.

Syringes with a lock device should not be used. This usually consists of a threaded needle attachment that requires that the needle be screwed onto or off of the syringe. In FNA, the only practical consequence of this device is that it slows removal of the needle and slightly delays specimen processing. Scanty specimens may dry slightly during this period, and bloody material may clot. Either can yield suboptimal results when the material is studied at the microscope. Furthermore, the risk of needle-stick injury and its infectious consequences increases as manipulation of the needle increases.

## Syringe Holder

In most situations, we use the metal syringe holder shown in Figure 1.3. An exception to its use is when performing aspiration without suction, discussed subsequently in this chapter (i.e., the Zajdela technique). The metal syringe holder is preferred over its plastic imitations and weighs only 190 grams. Such devices are usually available in two sizes, which accommodate either a 10-cc or a 20-cc syringe. As mentioned earlier, we prefer the 10-cc or 12-cc size, while some authors are completely at home with the larger apparatus.

The reason for using the syringe holder is that it permits both the needle placement and the syringe's application and release of suction to be accom-

Figure 1.3.
*Metal pistol-grip syringe holder for FNA procedures: Illustrated here is the 10-cc size, shown with a 12-cc syringe and a 25-gauge needle of 1½-inch (38 mm) length.*

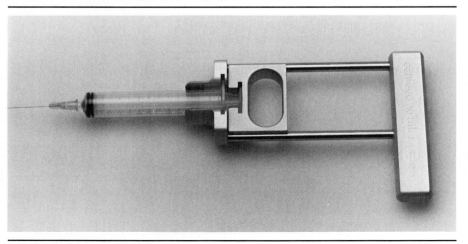

plished with one hand. Suction is not applied until after the needle is within the mass being studied and is released before the needle is withdrawn. Because of this, suction in the syringe is sufficient to return the plunger to its neutral position at the conclusion of the aspiration. Therefore, this action is automatic, requiring no additional effort by the physician performing the aspiration.

When the apparatus shown in Figure 1.3 is assembled, it can be held as shown in Figure 1.4. This arrangement affords an unbroken straight line, directly linking the physician's most accurate localizing tool—the index finger—and the needle tip that must be placed in the lesion to be studied.

As is apparent, the other hand (usually the left) is completely free. As shown in Figure 1.5, this hand can locate and stabilize the target lesion. Various techniques by which this can be accomplished optimally are discussed in Chapter 2. The most common arrangement is that shown in Figure 1.5, in which the index and second fingers stabilize the palpable mass.

Some prefer not to use any sort of syringe holder. If one hand is to be left free to stabilize the target, the other must both hold the syringe and manipulate the plunger, as shown in Figure 1.6. When full negative pressure is developed, a considerable amount of strength is required of the fingers. The effort thus demanded of the small intrinsic muscles of the hand robs it of the supple control of very fine movements, which is its forte. Furthermore, comparison of Figures 1.5 and 1.6 shows that without the syringe holder, the physician is aiming, not with the index finger, but with the thumb or with the hand as a whole. Thus, the opportunity to make the needle an extension of the index finger is lost.

Figure 1.4.
*Right-hand grip of the syringe-holder apparatus. A continuous straight line is formed by the index finger, the syringe barrel, and the needle.*

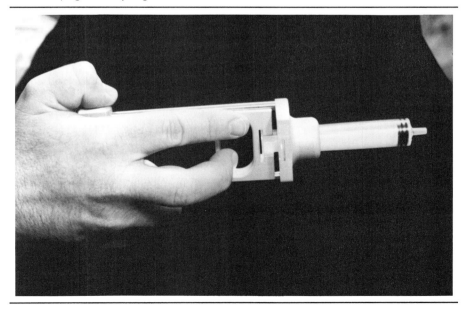

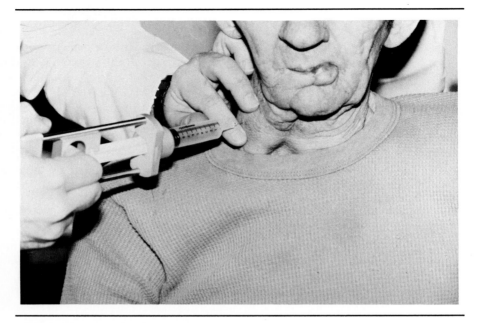

Figure 1.5.
*The basic position employed for aspiration of a palpable mass: The right hand operates the syringe holder, while the left hand is free to locate and stabilize the target lesion. In this case, the mass under study is a cervical lymph-node metastasis from a previously resected floor-of-mouth squamous-cell carcinoma. (Photograph reprinted from* The Oxford Textbook of Pathology, *Section 30.5, by permission of Oxford University Press, 1992.)*

Manufacturers of medical equipment occasionally market new FNA syringe holders or other devices. In general, these seem to us to present no meaningful advance over the instrument already described. When compared to various plastic holders, the metal holder represents a larger initial cost, but will probably outlast the professional career of its purchaser.

Sterile, plastic, disposable syringe holders are now available (Lee Medical Ltd., Syringe Division, Minneapolis, Minnesota). We do not employ such instruments in our daily clinic practice. However, such holders should enjoy considerable utility in the surgical suite, where they afford a simple means for surgeons to perform intraoperative FNA. Surgeons trained in bedside FNA and accustomed to using a syringe pistol will welcome this device. Alternatively, the standard metal instrument can be sterilized for use in the surgical suite.

## QUANTITY OF TISSUE OBTAINED BY FINE-NEEDLE ASPIRATION

For those unacquainted with this procedure, the first objection to diagnosis of tumors by aspiration with small-gauge needles is that the technique could not possibly yield enough tissue for meaningful diagnosis. These individuals seem to feel that the specimens obtained must be a small and inherently inferior substitute

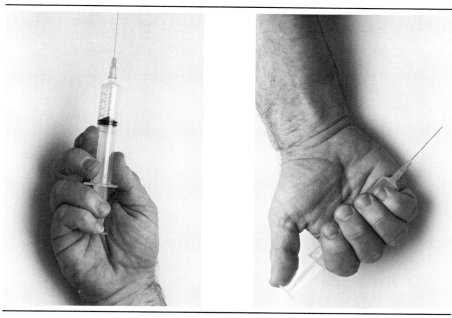

Figure 1.6.
*The alternative to using a syringe holder is to both hold the syringe and manipulate the plunger, using only one hand. Each of the two techniques shown here causes tension in the hand and lessens the practitioner's ability to carefully aim the needle as an extension of the index finger. Although suitable for large targets, such methods may not suffice for accurate puncture of very small lesions.*

for surgical biopsy. The accumulated evidence of the illustrations in this book reflect an attempt to dispel this belief. In fact, FNA often provides very generous tissue sampling. The tissue obtained is often more abundant than that in well-accepted biopsy methods, such as transbronchial biopsy, endoscopic bowel biopsy, or cutting-needle-core biopsy. Though qualitatively different, FNA specimens are often quantitatively superior to methods for biopsy of solid tissue fragments. For the present, four typical examples illustrate the abundance of tissue that can be obtained with this method, using 25-gauge needles: (1) breast tissue, (2) thyroid masses, (3) porotid-gland tumor, and (4) malignant melanoma. Additional examples can be found in Chapter 3.

When benign breast tissue is aspirated, a typical smear may include adipose tissue, fibrous tissue, ductal cell groups, myoepithelial cells, and lobular tissue, in varying proportions. Figure 1.7 shows an entire mammary lobule composed of multiple secretory units. Aspiration of benign thyroid masses may yield entire macrofollicles; a typical example, shown in Figure 1.8, is centrally filled with colloid. Figure 1.9 shows a smear from a benign mixed tumor (pleomorphic adenoma), the most frequently aspirated neoplasm of the parotid gland. Its most characteristic feature is extracellular matrix material that is chondroid in appearance. Numerous large tissue fragments are readily visible in this low-magnification image. The amount of tissue and even the size of tissue fragments

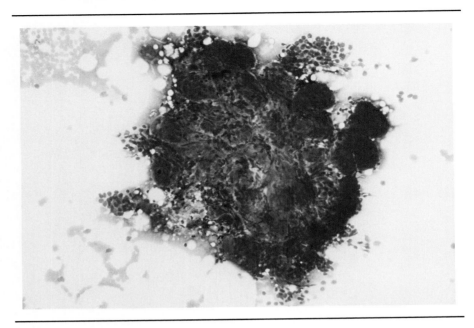

Figure 1.7.
*An entire lobule of benign breast tissue is seen here, as it was aspirated, using a 25-gauge needle (modified Diff-Quik® stain, magnification ×60 before a 28% reduction).*

Figure 1.8.
*A complete thyroid macrofollicle, formed by many cells and filled centrally with colloid, was aspirated from a benign nodular hyperplasia (colloid nodule) (Papanicolaou stain, magnification ×312 before a 28% reduction).*

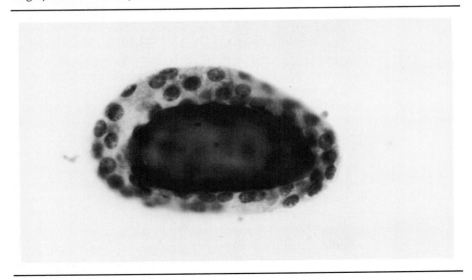

is greater than that sometimes obtained by endoscopic biopsy procedures, which are submitted for examination by the pathologist. Not all aspirations of tumors yield large tissue fragments such as those in Figure 1.9; sometimes, instead, large numbers of poorly cohesive cells may be present without forming particles large enough to be visible to the naked eye. One such case is depicted microscopically in Figure 1.10.

FNA selectively removes tumor cells of carcinoma, melanoma, or lymphoma. Much of the connective tissue is left behind. The result is concentration of the diagnostic cells of interest. Thus, FNA often gives better sampling than do biopsy methods that appear to remove larger pieces of tissue. With biopsy methods, much of the tissue may be stroma rather than tumor cells.

As illustrated briefly with Figures 1.7 through 1.10, properly performed aspiration with 25-gauge needles can yield large amounts of well-preserved tissue suitable for accurate diagnosis of many benign and malignant masses. Further illustration of this fact is provided as specific techniques, applications, and examples of FNA are considered (see Chapter 2). Issues of specimen adequacy are discussed in Chapter 3.

Figure 1.9.
*This smear from a benign mixed tumor (pleomorphic adenoma) of the parotid shows many large tissue fragments (modified Diff-Quik® stain, magnification ×60 before a 34% reduction).*

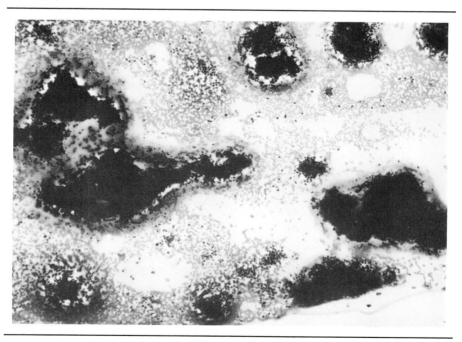

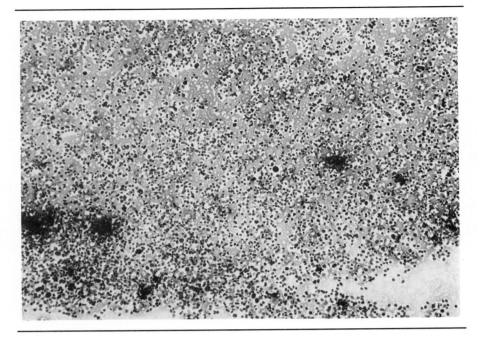

Figure 1.10.
*This very cellular smear is from a case of malignant melanoma. While these malignant cells are not sufficiently cohesive to form tissue fragments visible to the naked eye, a large total amount of tissue is present. This photomicrograph shows one of many such fields on one of five smears made from one aspiration with a 25-gauge needle (modified Diff-Quik® stain, magnification ×60 before a 34% reduction).*

## BASIC TECHNIQUES IN FINE-NEEDLE ASPIRATION

### The Aspiration Procedure

As noted previously, FNA can be adapted to many clinical settings and problems, but the basic procedure is constant throughout. While the total number of punctures performed on a given patient varies with the clinical situation, we usually say that each aspiration takes about 5 to 10 seconds. Additional time is spent examining the lesion, preparing the skin, and processing the material obtained by FNA, but the actual aspiration event is very brief. Despite the procedure's simplicity, we recommend that new practitioners gain practice implementing the procedure smoothly, quickly, and in an atraumatic way. We usually introduce the basic motions to new practitioners using an inanimate patient. Our usual surrogate is a piece of fruit.

For the moment, we set aside such important issues as patient positioning, physical examination, and smear preparation, as we concentrate on the basic process of performing the aspiration. This is illustrated in a stepwise fashion in Figures 1.11 through 1.16 and is summarized in Table 1.3.

Table 1.3
*Summary of the steps involved in the basic fine-needle aspiration procedure*

| Aspiration Procedure Step | Suction Applied | Illustration (Figure number) |
|---|---|---|
| 1. Locate, palpate, and stabilize the target lesion | | 1.5, 1.11 |
| 2. Pass the needle through the skin | No | 1.12 |
| 3. Advance the needle into the lesion | No | |
| 4. Apply suction | Yes | 1.13 |
| 5. Move the needle repeatedly through the mass, in various directions | Yes | 1.14 |
| 6. Release suction | No | |
| 7. Remove the needle from the patient | No | |
| 8. Detach the needle from the syringe | | |
| 9. Fill the syringe with air | | |
| 10. Replace the needle onto the syringe | | |
| 11. Change the grip on the syringe holder | | 1.15 |
| 12. Touch the needle tip to a microscope slide | | 1.16 |
| 13. Express the specimen onto the microscope slide | | 1.16 |
| 14. Prepare the smears | | |
| 15. Fix or dry the smears | | |

The initial step is localization of the mass to be punctured. Even at this early stage in our consideration of clinical methods, it is important to emphasize the need for delicacy and control. Large targets can be successfully (if inelegantly) punctured by any technique, however crude or impractical. However, many masses that can be successfully studied by FNA are quite small, and only a controlled approach with studied technique will suffice.

As shown in Figure 1.11, two fingers of the nondominant (usually the left) hand outline and immobilize the mass under study. In the case of large tumors, only a portion of the mass is spanned by the fingertips. In smaller masses, the entire tumor is frequently encompassed by this method. In addition to localizing the lesion, this approach allows the aspirator to apply pressure to the mass to form a fixed, immobile target at which to aim the needle, even with a very mobile tumor (such as a breast fibroadenoma). In all cases, the fingers are arched and extend from the hand, which is poised above a point near the palpable mass. As shown in Figure 1.11, this makes use of the sensitive fingertips in localizing the intended site of puncture. Furthermore, in this position, the small intrinsic muscles of the hand are relaxed. In this way, the very fine movements of the fingertips may help to ensure accurate puncture of small masses. Many of these techniques are discussed more fully in Chapter 2, when aspiration of breast masses is considered.

Once the mass has been localized and stabilized, the syringe holder can now be taken up with the grip shown in Figure 1.4. The needle can then be passed through the skin en route to the lesion. Figure 1.12 illustrates that so far, no suction has been applied.

At this point, the mental and physical process of ensuring that the needle tip actually enters the mass begins. Various aids to accomplishing this goal are described in Chapter 2. For now, it is useful to begin thinking of the needle as an

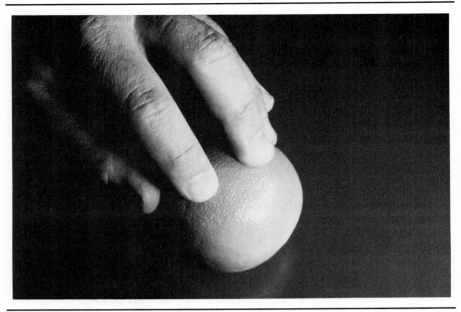

Figure 1.11.
*The mass is localized and held stable between the index and middle fingers of the nondominant (usually the left) hand. The fingers are arched, and the hand is poised above the mass so that the sensitive fingertips are employed. (Photograph reprinted from* The Oxford Textbook of Pathology, *Section 30.5, by permission of Oxford University Press, 1992.)*

Figure 1.12.
*The needle is first passed through the skin en route to the mass to be sampled. No suction has been applied. (Photograph reprinted from* The Oxford Textbook of Pathology, *Section 30.5, by permission of Oxford University Press, 1992.)*

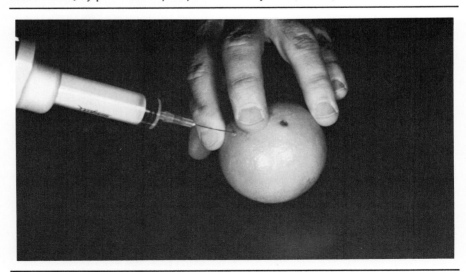

extension of the dominant (usually the right) hand's index finger and the mass as an extension of the palpating fingers of the nondominant hand. Thus, the sometimes difficult task of hitting a small target resembles touching the tip of one index finger with the other. This concept creates the possibility of subtle nuances of touch and pressure between the needle and the mass. Such delicacy and control are essential if small lesions are to be well sampled consistently.

At this time, the needle is advanced into the lesion, and then suction is applied (Figure 1.13). Next begins the process that is probably responsible for the generous sampling with very thin needles that is the hallmark of FNA. The needle is moved back and forth through the mass, in different directions, using a sewing-machine-like motion. Suction is maintained throughout this process. This activity fills the several seconds that are required for the typical aspiration. By this method, the needle can cut loose many small pieces of tissue that are then aspirated due to the suction applied by the syringe. The actual motion causes the needle tip to describe a cone, with its base in or near the mass and its apex at the point where the needle enters the skin, as shown in Figure 1.14.

In Chapters 2 and 3, we illustrate the quantitative aspects of material that can be obtained by aspiration of various body sites. This will include decisions about how many separate punctures are needed to address particular clinical issues. In general, most aspirations are terminated when material begins to appear in the needle hub. This area is monitored for material during the aspiration procedure. In some instances, larger volumes of either cyst fluid or blood may be obtained.

Figure 1.13.
*The needle is advanced into the lesion, and then suction is applied. (Photograph reprinted from* The Oxford Textbook of Pathology, *Section 30.5, by permission of Oxford University Press, 1992.)*

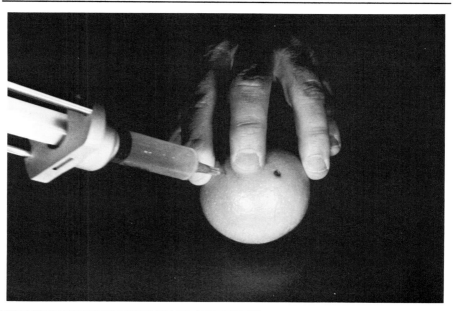

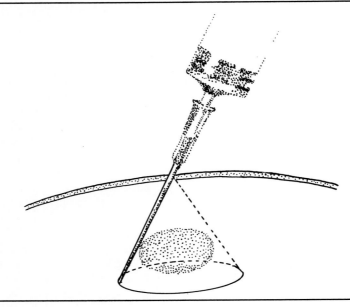

Figure 1.14.
*The needle is moved back and forth through the mass in different directions. Its tip describes a cone-shaped volume of sampled tissue, with its base near the mass and its apex at the skin surface. (Photograph reprinted from* The Oxford Textbook of Pathology, *Section 30.5, by permission of Oxford University Press, 1992.)*

As noted in Chapter 2, the practitioner must maintain a split focus of vision, both to monitor the needle hub and to evaluate the patient's face for evidence of distress during FNA.

The steps taken up to this point have been centered on ensuring an accurate puncture of even small palpable masses and on securing a diagnostically effective sample. The next step is designed to protect the specimen that has been obtained. All suction is released, by allowing the syringe plunger to return gently to its resting position. Because the needle is still in the mass (or at least under the skin surface), the negative pressure within the syringe will cause this to happen without any effort from the physician except relaxation of the fingers that have been pulling back on the plunger.

At this point in the procedure, most or all of the specimen is in the needle itself, though a small amount may be in the needle hub. Except in the case of cyst fluids, very bloody aspirations, or high-volume specimens such as may be seen in the aspiration of an abscess or an area of necrosis, little or no material will be in the syringe itself. The purpose of releasing suction before the needle is withdrawn is to leave the aspirated material largely in the needle. If the needle is withdrawn with suction still applied, the specimen is drawn quickly into the syringe, during which time, it breaks up into numerous small droplets. These in turn are deposited forcefully onto the walls of the syringe barrel where they are quickly desiccated and virtually impossible to recover intact. The vital importance of releasing suction before withdrawing the syringe was well illustrated by the study of Furnival et al. By addition of this simple suction-release step to their aspiration protocol, these authors reduced the rate of unsatisfactory breast aspiration from 24.8 percent to 6 percent (total series = 237 cases).[5]

Once the suction is released, the needle is withdrawn from the patient. While continuing not to apply suction to the syringe, the needle is detached from the syringe. (The specimen is still in the needle and its hub.) While the needle is detached, the syringe is filled with air. Next, the needle, with its specimen, can be replaced onto the syringe. The air in the syringe is used to gently expel the specimen onto a glass microscope slide. We find it comfortable and efficient to use a different grip on the syringe pistol at this point, as shown in Figure 1.15; it is held like a syringe being used for an injection. During this procedure, the needle should be held firmly onto the syringe with the nondominant hand. If the needle is not held tightly attached to the syringe as the sample is expelled, and if the specimen is thick or clotted, the needle may fly forcefully from the syringe.

When the specimen is placed on the slide, we prefer to keep the needle tip in actual contact with the surface of the slide, usually with the bevel at a 45° to 90° angle to the slide's surface (Figure 1.16). If, instead, the specimen is allowed to spray or drop onto the slide from a needle held above the slide, the impact causes the specimen to break up into droplets that are rapidly dried as they spread out on the slide's surface. Figure 1.17 shows the results of such a spraying of the specimen. Contrast this with the small concentrated droplet in Figure 1.16.

Figure 1.15.
*A different grip on the syringe pistol is used for carefully controlling the expression of aspirated material onto a glass microscope slide. The nondominant hand stabilizes and holds the needle firmly attached to the syringe.*

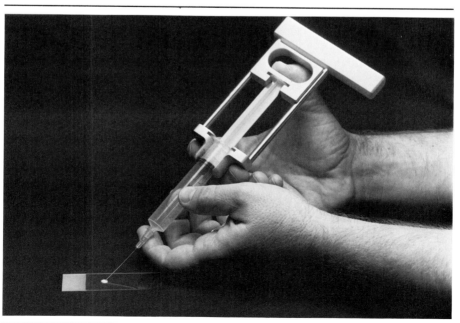

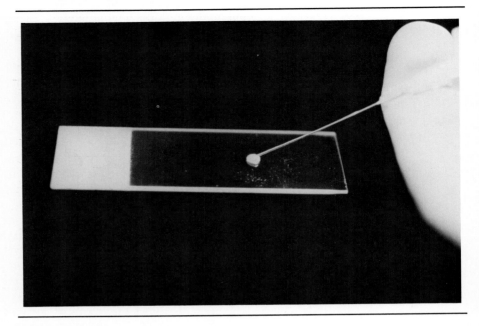

Figure 1.16.
*The specimen is gently expressed onto the slide's surface. The needle bevel is held at an angle of 45° to 90° from the slide surface, and the needle tip touches the slide. Specimens of the type shown here form a small droplet.*

Specimen desiccation is virtually nonexistent in the small droplet. Furthermore, if a moment or two is needed to attend to the patient prior to attending to the specimen, cytologic integrity will not be lost by allowing the specimen to rest briefly in its tissue fluid. The aspirated material can be stored briefly, either within the needle or as a small droplet on the glass slide.

## Zajdela Technique

In many instances, capillary action without aspiration will suffice to admit cells and tissue particles into a thin needle. This is the basis of the technique described by Zajdela et al.[6] In this method, the mass is localized and stabilized with the fingers of the nondominant hand, as previously described. The thin needle of appropriate length is held by the dominant hand thumb, index finger, and middle finger; the grip is very much like that used to hold a pencil. After the needle is advanced into the lesion, it is moved about in a cone-shaped tissue volume similar to that discussed earlier (see Figure 1.14). It is then withdrawn. A syringe filled with air is attached and is used to expel the specimen onto a microscope slide, for smear preparation.

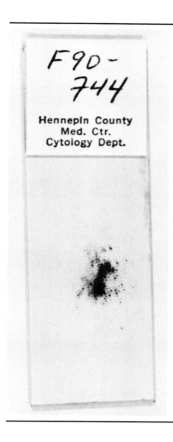

Figure 1.17.
*This slide shows the typical appearance of a specimen
having been sprayed onto its surface from above,
rather than having been gently placed, as in Figure
1.16. The central portion of the specimen is too
thick for microscopic study, while the small droplets
will show poor quality, due to rapid dessication.*

We have found this method most useful for very small lesions. The needle grip described in the preceding paragraph gives excellent control. It also gives the physician an extraordinary degree of sensitivity to changes in the texture of tissues through which the needle passes. These benefits improve the practitioner's ability to puncture certain tiny masses. Zajdela et al. describe successful application of this method to study of small masses around the eye, including those in the lids.[6]

It has been suggested that adding aspiration (that is, performing FNA in the traditional manner) lowers the rate of inadequate sampling when benign breast masses are studied.[7] This probably reflects the fact that many of these masses consist largely of fibrofatty tissue and yield sparsely cellular samples under the best of circumstances. (The very important sampling issues in breast cytology are discussed more fully in Chapter 2.)

In our experience, the Zajdela method yields fewer cells than aspiration, but it provides sufficient material for diagnosis of most lesions. The needle can be concealed in the palm of the physician's hand, and the patient is spared seeing the large syringe and syringe holder that some find alarming. Thus, patients are very accepting of this technique.

## Preparation of Smears

### Comments on Technical Assistance during FNA

As we open this section on technical handling of aspirated material, we wish to comment on a situation that is common in North America but is not often seen in Sweden. In Sweden, most FNA is in the hands of a single individual who is a clinician–cytopathologist, who examines the patient, reviews the medical record, performs the aspiration, prepares the material, examines the smears, and reports the results. While the authors feel that this is the best way to perform FNA, we acknowledge that there are many settings in which the aspirator and the microscopist are not the same individual. In our experience, this situation often produces poor-quality specimens. An exception to this is the institution in which a small number of experienced clinicians perform aspirations frequently and produce excellent results by working closely with a small number of microscopists. Those clinicians who only occasionally use FNA seldom achieve success in the technique. Certainly, those clinicians trained in the basic techniques of specimen preparation often perform the procedure well and send diagnostically useful material to the laboratory. However, a more frequent situation is that once obtained, the specimen is handed to a nurse, a student, or a resident physician who has no idea what to do with it. Thus, diagnostic material is converted to useless clots and crushed cells.

This situation can be ameliorated considerably by replacing the untrained nurse, student, or resident with a technically adept laboratory specialist. In the United States, this is usually a cytotechnologist. While many laboratories find it necessary to offer this service, one of its main effects is that it takes highly skilled laboratory personnel away from important work to spend time walking to the clinic or ward, and then waiting while patients are examined, charts are found, materials are located, and test requests are completed. This contributes to increased costs for all activities in that laboratory. As the nationwide shortage of cytotechnologists worsens, and as these skilled individuals command greater salaries, it may become increasingly difficult to offer this kind of service to clinicians. Thus, physicians wishing to perform FNA should take the time to master the entire procedure, including the specimen preparation.

Finally, some examples of improperly prepared material are shown in Figures 1.18 through 1.21. All are actual patient material sent to our laboratory.

### Glass Slides

The common type of glass slide in routine use measures 75 mm × 25 mm × 1 mm. An important consideration is slide labeling at the time of the procedure. Permanent labels with the laboratory's case accession number are affixed later. Labeling at the bedside should be rapid, convenient, and indelible. Most laboratories use two identifiers on each slide, such as the patient's name (or initials) and the site of the aspiration. We prefer slides that have one end frosted on both top and bottom sides of the slide surface. This frosted surface is very easy to write on with a pencil.

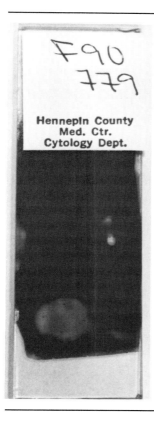

Figure 1.18.
*While otherwise a reasonable smear, the material on this slide is too thick for proper examination. Some cells at the very edge can be studied, but most of its material will not transmit light.*

We label slides at the bedside just before performing the aspiration, to minimize any possibility of confusing the material obtained from different patients. In processing the smears after staining, it will be important to apply a coverslip to the correct side of the slide and to be sure not to wipe the aspirated material from the surface as the slide is dried with gauze. By writing on the label and always applying smears to the same side as the label, no confusion over which side of the slide holds the specimen should occur. Scanty specimens may be difficult to identify by gross inspection of the slide, so that some such method is important, to ensure that no specimens will be lost while the slide is handled during processing.

For this purpose, we regard the frosted label as the top of the slide because it protrudes above the surface of liquid in the staining dishes during processing. It is inevitable that while labeling blank slides, one's hand will rest on the glass surface. If one tries to avoid this by inverting the slide for labeling, this results in an upside-down label that may negate the advantage just discussed.

Various substances have been used to increase the adherence of specimens to the slide surface. This is most important when using histologic sections of

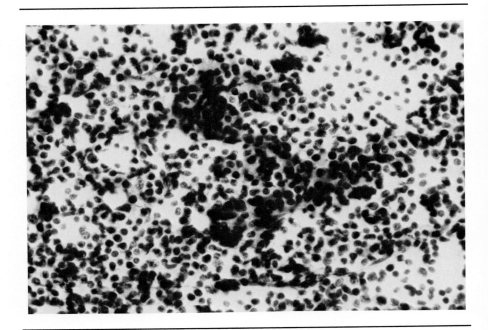

Figure 1.19.
*The microscopic appearance of the smear shown in Figure 1.18 is illustrated here. Multiple layers of cells are too crowded for detailed examination. Others appear damaged.*

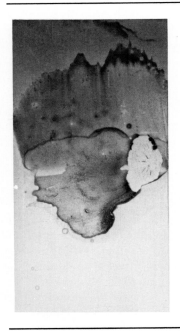

Figure 1.20.
*This smear consists largely of clotted blood. Such clots are often poorly adherent to the slide's surface. As illustrated here, part of the specimen has simply fallen off before coverslipping. Extensively clotted material is best prepared as a cell block for histologic study. (Photograph courtesy of Charles A. Horwitz, Metropolitan—Mt. Sinai Hospital, Minneapolis, Minnesota.)*

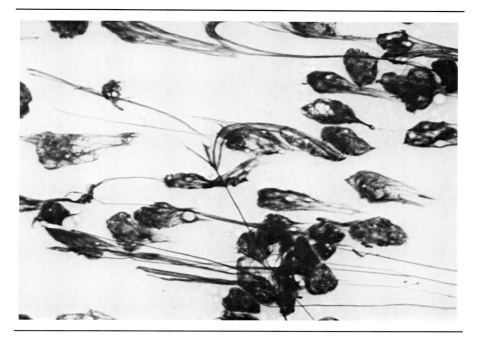

Figure 1.21.
*The cells on this slide have been crushed by too much pressure exerted during smearing.*
*Thus, the nature of such cells is unclear.*

paraffin-embedded tissue, especially during complex immunohistochemical procedures. The most commonly used adherents are alum, albumin, and polylysine. We have found these unnecessary for general FNA work and prefer to use uncoated slides, just as they come from the manufacturer's package. Another means of enhancing adherence is to use a slide on which the entire surface is frosted. These are not readily available in some clinics. Again, we find such aids unnecessary.

### Introduction to Smear Preparation

Although a variety of special studies can be applied to aspiration specimens, most specimens are spread on a glass slide, to form a smear suitable for routine light microscopy. We examine four ways of accomplishing this goal: (1) two-slide-pull method, (2) one-step method, (3) two-step method, and (4) modified two-step method. In each case, the object is the same. Cells are to be spread over the slide surface, ideally in a monolayer. Some tissue fragments will need to be spread apart with gentle pressure, and some will remain intact. While accomplishing these goals, the pressure applied to the specimen must not be so great as to crush the cells. The end result should be a smear with well-preserved cells, spread thinly enough to permit the transmission of light.

Selection of a smearing technique is dictated to some extent by the skills and preferences of the individual preparing the specimen. The physical properties of the specimen must also be considered; it is helpful to tailor the method to the

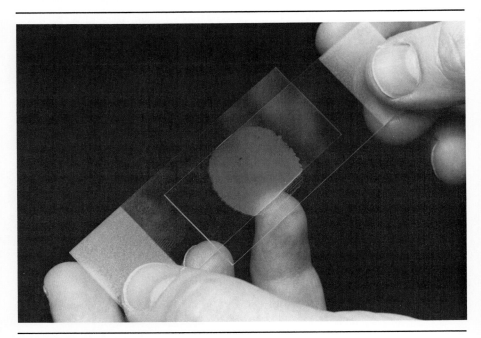

Figure 1.22.
*The two-slide-pull method of making a smear: A small droplet-sized portion of the specimen is spread between two slides.*

specimen, so that the best results are achieved. For example, a small droplet of semisolid tissue requires a different approach than that used for more fluid materials. In Chapters 2 and 3, we discuss the types of specimens obtained in some common clinical situations.

Many of the slides we illustrate have most or all of the specimen concentrated in a small area. These can be reviewed microscopically much more quickly than poorly made smears that do not concentrate tissue particles and that cover most of the slide surface. In our practice, most FNA smears do not require screening as do other preparations, such as gynecologic smears and sputum smears. This contributes to the rapid availability of results that is so highly valued in clinical practice, and it improves efficiency within the laboratory.

Preparation of aspirated material (usually in the form of smears) is one of the most important parts of the entire process. Unless high-quality preparations are created, it does not matter how adroit the aspiration or how skilled the microscopist; the material will be uninterpretable. Most alternatives to smear preparation introduce delays and increased costs.

### Two-Slide-Pull Method

The two-slide-pull method is widely used and is easy to learn. It is most useful with specimens of low volume. The specimen, or a small droplet-sized portion thereof, is placed near the center of the slide, as shown previously in Figure 1.16. A second, clean, previously labeled slide is inverted over the first, and gentle pressure is then applied, after which the two slides are slid apart, as in Figure 1.22. Both slides hold material, and both should be further processed. (The upper or spreader slide holds the specimen on its lower face and must be inverted before it is set aside for processing.)

If the specimen volume is too large, if excessive pressure is used in spreading the material, or if the droplet is placed too near the end of the slide, the resultant smear will look like that illustrated in Figure 1.23. In this example, much of the material has been carried to the very end of the slide, where it forms a dense zone that is too thick for careful microscopic study. The microscopic image of Figure 1.23 is shown in Figure 1.24.

### One-Step Method

We find that the one-step method produces high-quality smears. It is an excellent method for small-volume specimens. We prefer this technique to the two-slide-pull method because it allows precise control of the pressure applied to the specimen. Furthermore, it usually produces a smear that occupies a small area on the slide, thus facilitating rapid microscopic review.

In preparing to execute the maneuver, we hold the slides as shown in Figure 1.25. The lower slide holds the specimen and is held in the nondominant hand. With this grip, the slide is securely supported, but virtually its entire surface is free and available for the smear to be made. The upper slide is a spreader slide. When

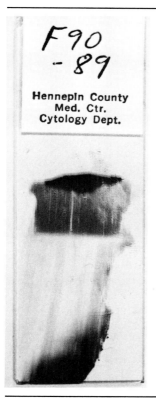

F90 -89

**Hennepin County Med. Ctr. Cytology Dept.**

Figure 1.23.
*Smears made by the two-slide-pull method: In this example, the specimen had been spread over too large an area, either by excessive pressure or by beginning with a specimen of too large a volume. Much of the material is collected at the very end of the slide, where it is too thick for proper examination.*

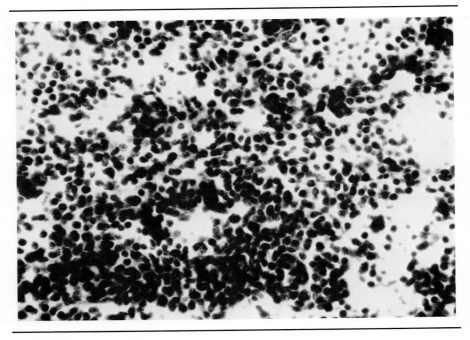

Figure 1.24.
*Microscopic view of the end of the smear shown in Figure 1.23: The cells are piled too thickly for proper examination. The cellular details are not visible (modified Diff-Quik® stain, magnification ×160 before a 34% reduction).*

using this technique, we place the specimen near the label at the upper edge of the slide. Thus, most of the slide's length is available for the smear.

The spreader slide is held at an angle so that its edge near the specimen is poised above the droplet, and its other edge touches the lower slide in a hingelike fashion. The far edge of the spreader slide is then lowered onto the droplet, as in Figure 1.26. Gentle pressure is applied to flatten but not crush the droplet. The spreader slide is then drawn along the length of the lower slide by pulling it toward the preparer. The pressure applied to the lower slide must be constant and gentle.

During this drawing out of the smear, the rectangular sides of the slide are perpendicular, but the flat surfaces of the two slides are parallel. It is important that the spreader slide not be tilted to either side of parallel. If its edge away from the lower slide's label is tilting toward the lower slide, the pressure on the specimen is decreased, and the smear will be too thick. If the edge near the label is tilted down, the specimen will be scraped off of the lower slide onto the edge of the spreader slide, where it forms a thick line from which diagnostic material is difficult to recover. With this method, very little material will be found on the spreader slide. We generally discard this, along with the needle used to perform the aspiration. A typical smear prepared in this manner is shown in Figure 1.27.

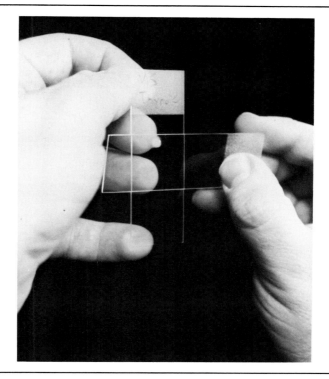

Figure 1.25.
*In preparing smears by the direct one-step technique, we hold the slide as shown here. The lower slide (in the nondominant hand) holds the specimen, while the upper slide (in the dominant hand) is used as a spreader slide. The spreader slide is perpendicular to the lower slide. The acute angle between the two slides always opens away from the individual holding the slides. The spreader slide is poised over the specimen droplet, with its lower edge forming a hingelike contact with the lower slide.*

### The Two-Step Method

The two-step method is tailored to liquid specimens. It is designed to handle a few drops of material (blood or other fluid) at a time. Cells or tissue particles (microscopic or macroscopic size) are suspended in the fluid. This method is illustrated in a stepwise fashion with Figures 1.28 through 1.34.

First, the fluid specimen is placed near the labeled end of the slide (Figure 1.28). Using the grip shown in Figure 1.22, the spreader slide is held at a 45° angle to the specimen-bearing slide, and its end is brought into contact with the lower slide in front of the specimen (Figure 1.29). It is then advanced until it just touches the specimen pool. Surface tension will cause the liquid to spread out in a line behind the edge of the spreader slide (Figure 1.30). The tissue particles will be carried with the fluid and are thus concentrated in a narrow band across the slide.

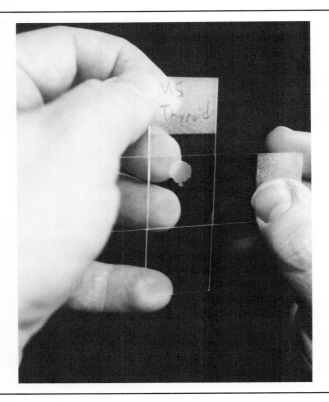

Figure 1.26.
*The top, far edge of the spreader slide is lowered onto the specimen droplet, and gentle pressure is used to flatten the specimen.*

Figure 1.27.
*A typical smear produced by the one-step method is shown. This is best applied to small-volume specimens. Small tissue particles are visible.*

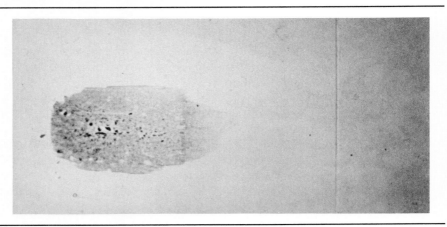

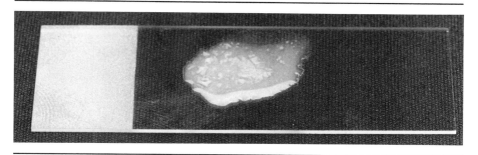

Figure 1.28.
*A typical specimen suitable for the two-step smear method: This drop of blood or other fluid containing cells or tissue particles is placed near the label end of a slide.*

Figure 1.29.
*The end of the spreader slide is touched to the specimen slide at a 45° angle.*

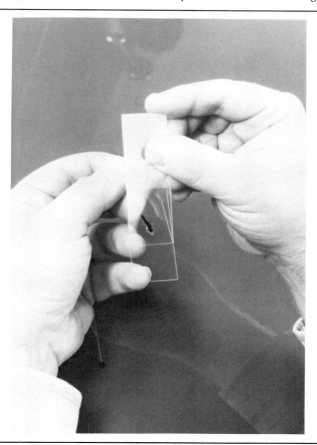

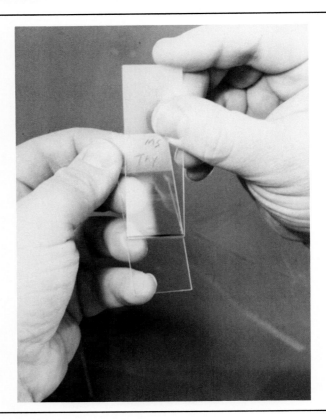

Figure 1.30.
*When the spreader slide is brought into contact with the specimen, the fluid spreads out along its edge. Tissue particles are distributed along this line.*

The spreader slide is then slid away from the specimen slide's label, to about the middle of the lower slide. At this point, the two slides are tilted together as a unit, so that the label ends point down. The spreader slide (which often bears some tissue at its distal end) is now quickly pulled away from the specimen slide. The spreader slide is retained in the dominant hand, while with the nondominant hand, the specimen slide is held vertically. The larger tissue particles are now sedimented along the line where the spreader slide was placed, and much of the fluid drains toward the label of the specimen slide and away from the tissue (Figure 1.31).

The procedure from this point on is very much like the one-step method described previously. The same spreader slide (still with tissue fragments on its distal end) is turned perpendicular to the specimen slide, and the line of tissue particles is smeared as before (Figure 1.32).

The tissue remaining on the distal end of the spreader slide must now be recovered. It can be placed either on the smear that has just been made (if there

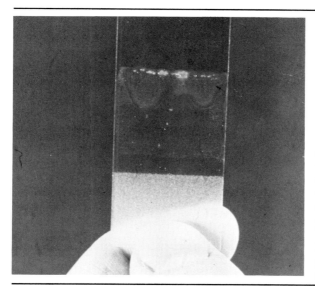

Figure 1.31.
*The spreader slide has been pulled away from the specimen slide and retained for later use. The specimen slide is held vertically, with its label pointing downward. The tissue particles are in a line at the middle of the slide, and much of the fluid now drains away toward the label end. (Photograph reprinted from* The Oxford Textbook of Pathology, *Section 30.5, by permission of Oxford University Press, 1992.)*

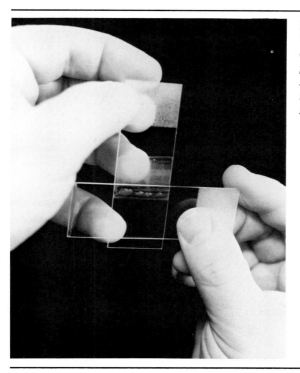

Figure 1.32.
*The spreader slide is now poised over the line of particles, as previously illustrated in the one-step method. Note that visible tissue remains on the end of the spreader slide.*

is additional room on that slide), or it can be put on a new slide. This method is demonstrated with a new slide in Figures 1.33 and 1.34. The spreader slide is touched to the new slide, near the label, at a 45° angle, with its line of fluid or tissue in the vertex of the angle. It is then lowered until it is parallel to the new specimen slide and drawn parallel to it, as in the two-slide-pull method. Figure 1.34 shows slides on which this spreader slide residual specimen has been added to a smear, such as that shown in Figure 1.32, and to one on which it has been added to a new slide, as that slide's only specimen.

The two-step method accomplishes two things: First, tissue particles are concentrated in a relatively small area of the slide for rapid viewing; second, much of the fluid has been removed from the diagnostically important part of the specimen. This permits either rapid, thorough fixation or rapid drying of the slide, whichever is preferred for the specimen at hand (each method is described subsequently in this chapter). The high-quality morphology of rapidly dried cells is totally lost if the cells are allowed to dry slowly in abundant fluid (see Figure 1.35). Slow drying damages the cells and causes them to appear exploded.

The two-step technique is more complex, but it greatly increases the number of specimens that can be smeared in a few seconds at the bedside. This is important because all the alternatives to rapidly made smears involve either centrifugation or histology-based embedding. In either case, specimen preparation is much slower and requires more time from laboratory personnel. Because

Figure 1.33.
*Tissue left on the end of the spreader slide is placed between it and the specimen slide. The spreader slide is brought parallel to the specimen slide. A smear can then be made as previously described in the two-slide-pull method. The slides are pulled apart, with their surfaces held constantly parallel.*

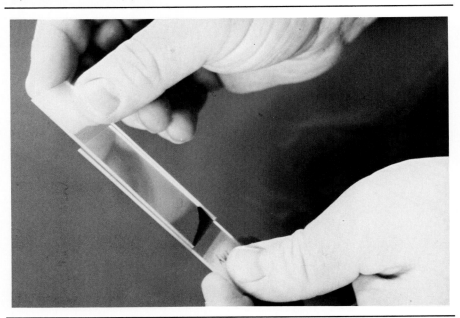

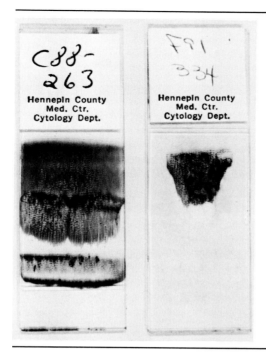

Figure 1.34.
*The spreader slide's residual tissue can be added to an already prepared two-step-method smear (left) or to a new slide (right). The smear on the left shows dark tissue fragments that occupy a small area of the slide. The blood shows the effect of running down when the slide was held vertically.*

Figure 1.35.
*Poorly prepared lung aspiration smear: The cells have dried very slowly in fluid and have a characteristic exploded appearance. Fluid-rich specimens with this type of artifact are unsuitable for interpretation (modified Diff- Quik® stain, magnification ×312 before a 34% reduction).*

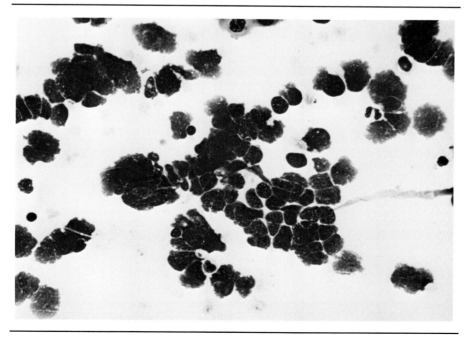

some of the chief advantages of FNA are its rapidity, simplicity, low cost, and lack of a need for highly skilled laboratory personnel, these alternative methods would reduce markedly its utility and attractiveness.

### Modified Two-Step Method

The modified two-step method has the same advantages as the two-step technique, but it is designed to handle a larger volume of blood or fluid, up to 0.5 cc per slide. Within a few seconds, most of the tissue particles will sediment. The slide can then be picked up and rotated gently. (This is much like panning for gold.) As the particles sediment over a large area of the slide, the fluid can be moved to the edge of the slide by this motion. Unless its volume is excessive, surface tension will keep the liquid on the slide. The slide is then tipped vertically, and the fluid is removed by bringing a piece of gauze to the edge of the slide. The gauze will act as a wick (Figure 1.36). Alternatively, this fluid can be removed with a small glass pipette with suction bulb attached and then processed by centrifugation for cytologic examination or special studies.

The particles on the slide must now be brought together. A spreader slide is touched to the specimen slide at a 45° angle (Figure 1.37). By drawing this slide toward the label of the specimen slide, the tissue is collected in a line similar to that previously described in the two-step method (Figure 1.38). A smear of this line is now made as previously illustrated (see Figure 1.32). The material on the end of the spreader slide can be recovered as shown in Figures 1.33 and 1.34. A

Figure 1.36.
*In the modified two-step method, the particles have been allowed to sediment, the fluid is moved to the slide's edge by rotating the slide, and the gauze acts as a wick to remove the fluid.*

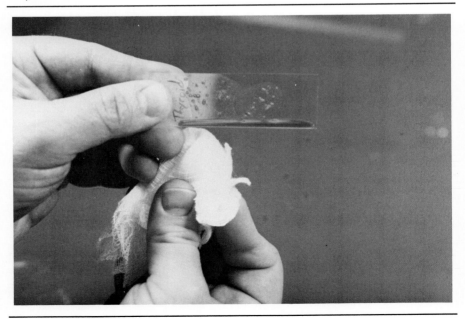

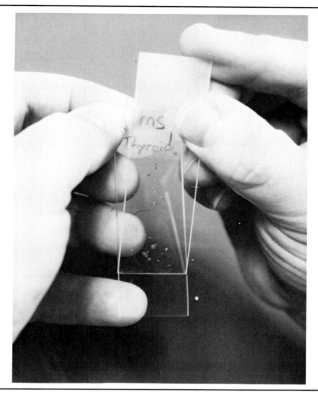

Figure 1.37.
*A clean spreader slide is now touched to the specimen slide at a 45° angle.*

smear prepared by the modified two-step method resembles one prepared by the two-step method.

## Alternative to Rapid Preparation of Smears

We now describe a final method for specimen preparation, which we rarely use in our own practice. The material obtained by aspiration can be expressed into a liquid fixative. Those that have been suggested include Saccomanno's fluid (2% Carbowax in 50% ethanol), 95 percent ethanol, and 50 percent methanol. Once received in the laboratory, this fluid is processed by laboratory personnel, using a centrifuge or membrane filtration.

The advantage of this method is obvious: When nonpathologists perform aspirations, this technique relieves them of any need to be able to make smears, and laboratory personnel are not required to attend to the preparation procedure. Furthermore, the specimen is preserved in a form suitable for transport to the laboratory.

Its disadvantages are several. The cost of FNA goes up when laboratory processing is added. Furthermore, the turnaround time for such material is longer than that for smears made at the time of aspiration. In the hospital setting, or in the clinic attached to the hospital, many smears can be stained, examined,

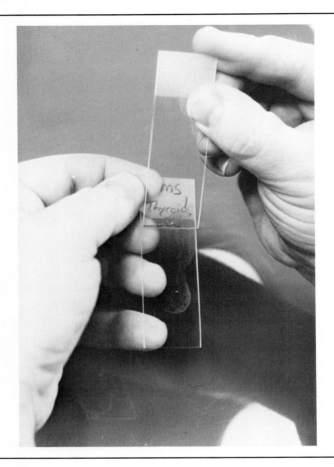

Figure 1.38.
*As the spreader slide is drawn toward the label of the specimen slide, the tissue particles collect in a line behind it.*

and reported in 30 minutes or less. For many clinicians, this is an important motivation for using FNA. Also, from the cytopathologists' point of view, having only fixed material limits the staining possibilities. Specifically, Romanowsky stains (the group of staining methods applied to air-dried smears, as in hematologic preparations) cannot be applied to fixed material. Some cytopathologists strongly prefer air-dried, Romanowsky-stained smears in many settings. (A more complete discussion of staining options and their importance is offered later in this chapter.)

### Preparation of Several Smears from a Single Aspiration

It is often the case, especially in the study of malignancies, that a single aspiration will give more material than is needed for one slide. Indeed, if too much material is placed on a single slide, it will be too thick for examination. We take advantage of this and distribute the material among the original specimen slide and one or more additional slides. We frequently have the experience of making four or more high-quality, richly cellular smears from one puncture of a malignant mass.

We begin by expressing the entire specimen onto a specimen slide, as shown previously (see Figure 1.16). The end of a spreader slide is now placed in the specimen pool at a 45° angle, as shown in Figure 1.39. This is then moved rapidly and smoothly to the edge of the specimen slide and carried off its edge. At this point, the original specimen slide has a portion of its material still in place, while the spreader slide bears tissue on its distal end (Figure 1.40). The material on the specimen slide is smeared with the spreader slide, as in the one-step method (Figures 1.26 and 1.27). The material on the end of the spreader slide can now be placed onto a new slide and smeared, as in Figures 1.33 and 1.34.

If the specimen on the end of the spreader slide is large enough, a small portion of it can be deposited on each of two or more slides by gently touching them with the specimen droplet. Each of the new specimen slides is then smeared by using the one-step method. In this way, several smears have been rapidly prepared from one aspiration. This opens up the possibility of having extra smears for special stains or other studies, as needed.

When the edge or corner of a spreader slide is gently touched to an expressed specimen droplet, a small amount will adhere to the spreader slide. It can then be transferred by touching it to a new specimen slide. In this way, many small smears can be prepared. In the case of highly cellular material, such as lymph

Figure 1.39.
*In preparing to split a generous specimen, the edge of a spreader slide is used to partition a specimen pool as shown.*

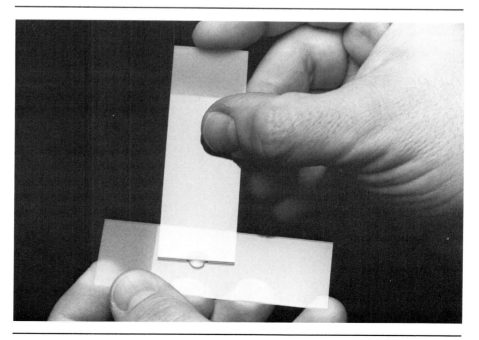

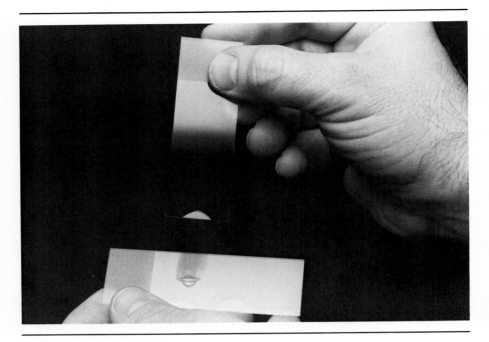

Figure 1.40.
*The spreader slide has been moved off the edge of the specimen slide and now holds tissue on its distal end. The original specimen slide still has a portion of its original material.*

node aspirations, these tiny smears may be thinner and better for microscopic examination than the thicker smears prepared from the entire specimen droplet or from large portions thereof.

These methods of splitting a specimen can also be applied to either the two-step or the modified two-step procedure. The spreader slide can be used to partition the line of tissue fragments that was produced early in these procedures (see Figures 1.31 and 1.38). The remaining portion of the line of tissue particles can then be smeared to yield a slide such as that illustrated in Figure 1.41.

It cannot be overemphasized that while the foregoing descriptions may seem tedious to the reader, they can be mastered with practice and are always executed within a few seconds. Just as the basic motions of the FNA procedure should be mastered before the patient is approached, so should the handling of aspirated material. Smear making can be practiced using droplets of lotion, liquid soap, or yogurt. The fluid-rich materials suitable for the two-step or modified two-step method can be simulated by material aspirated from an orange. Bloody or fluid-rich smears can also be practiced by aspirating a bit of liver from the butcher shop.

The motivation for going to all this bother is that this repertoire of techniques will greatly increase the number of specimens that can be rapidly and inexpensively handled by FNA. Also, the aspirated material is of optimum quality when smears are well made, the tissue is concentrated, and the fluid or blood is largely removed. Unstained smears can be stored or transported, as necessary. Table 1.4 presents a summary of the techniques for preparing microscopic smears.

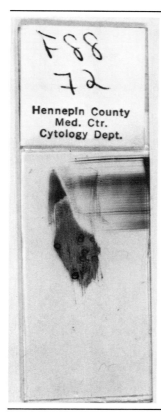

Figure 1.41.
*A smear made by the two-step method, from which part of the material has been removed for preparation of additional smears.*

Table 1.4
*Summary of techniques for preparation of microscopic smears*

| Smear Technique | Specimen Volume | Illustrations (Figure numbers) |
|---|---|---|
| Two-slide-pull method | Droplet | 1.18 to 1.20 |
| One-step method | Droplet | 1–21 to 1.23 |
| Two-step method | Fluid drops | 1.24 to 1.30 |
| Two-step method, modified for larger fluid volumes | Up to 0.5 cc | 1.32 to 1.34 |
| Expression into fixative for centrifugation* or filtration | Any type | |

*Centrifugation can be with a cytocentrifuge. Alternatively, the whole volume can be centrifuged, and smears can be prepared from the pellet, using one of the other methods.

## Clotting of Aspiration Specimens

Extremely bloody specimens are always suboptimal, but many can be improved considerably by use of the modified two-step smear technique. When clotting occurs, the material is unsuitable for cytologic examination and must be fixed (usually in formalin) and embedded for histologic study.

Some operators use heparinized syringes to reduce clotting. Those wishing to use this method should draw a small amount of heparin through the needle into the syringe. This should then be expelled as completely as possible. Tiny amounts are sufficient to impede clotting, but larger amounts will result in unwanted artifacts when cells are studied microscopically.

In general, we agree with Kung et al. that heparin is rarely necessary. These authors discussed liver FNA, which often yields bloody material. They indicate that by handling the material quickly, clotting does not occur before smears are prepared.[8]

## Embedded Cell Blocks (Histologic Preparation of Aspirated Material)

Occasional bloody specimens clot rapidly and completely. These are unsuitable for smears and for cytologic interpretation, leaving histologic study as the only alternative. In other cases, histologic material is desirable, in addition to cytologic preparations. In either of these instances, we place the aspirated material in a liquid fixative such as Bouin's or 10 percent neutral buffered formalin. This can be done by expressing the needle's contents directly into fluid (Figure 1.42). This is then centrifuged, and the pellet is embedded for sectioning as one handles any small-tissue biopsy.

If the clotted material is already on the surface of a slide, it can be collected, as in the modified two-step method (see Figures 1.37 and 1.38), and then

Figure 1.42.
*Material from an aspiration is expressed directly into a fixative. This can then be processed and sectioned for viewing as a histologic specimen.*

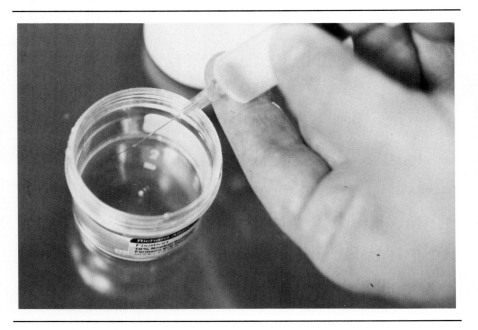

removed from the slide, as in splitting aspirated material (see Figures 1.39 and 1.40).

Bloody specimens can be expressed onto a slide and intentionally set aside briefly, to allow clotting. This material can then be placed in fixative solution. We use this method frequently (in addition to smear preparation) during radiographically directed aspirations when cell-block material is desirable (discussed subsequently herein). Material obtained by rinsing the needle and syringe is also suitable for preparation of cell blocks.

We find this cell-block method especially useful in preparing large numbers of tissue sections for immunohistochemistry (discussed subsequently herein). Other methods for preparing embedded histologic blocks from liquid specimens are described in the general literature of cytology. One or more of these methods are available in most laboratories. With any of these methods, overnight processing, with its inevitable delay, must be anticipated.

Because FNA of palpable masses is easily repeated, and because most cases do not require histologic material for diagnosis, we do not routinely prepare cell blocks in all cases. On the other hand, when material is obtained with radiographic guidance or by endoscopic means, repeating the procedure is difficult and costly and causes delays in patient care. In these settings, we often prepare cell blocks.

## Additional Techniques

An effort should be made to recover all of the aspirated material. Occasionally, volumes of nonclotting fluid greater than 0.5 cc are obtained. These are usually submitted to the cytology laboratory for centrifugation, after which the sedimented material is prepared by one of the smearing techniques previously described or as a fixed cell block for histologic study. Most of the time, however, smaller amounts of material are obtained.

At times, some of this aspirated material will be lodged in the hub of the needle or in the distal part of the syringe. Tissue fragments in the needle hub will never be recovered by repeated blasts of air from the syringe through the needle, no matter how forceful they may be. Instead, these particles can be deposited on a slide by holding the needle in the hand and then repeatedly and forcefully hitting the open end of the hub against the surface of the slide (Figure 1.43). Each of the authors has executed this maneuver several thousand times without incurring accidental needle-stick injury. Most individuals will want to practice this technique with unused sterile needles before applying it to needles containing potentially infectious patient material. The needle can also be gripped with a hemostat, to reduce the danger of an accidental needle-stick injury. Slides produced in this manner will hold a few or even several small fluid droplets. These can then be collected as in the modified two-step method, so that they form a line to be smeared with another slide. We have frequently observed that the material in the hub is the most diagnostic part of the specimen, the subsequently aspirated material having been contaminated with blood or fluid. Thus, recovery, smearing, and study of this portion of the specimen is very important.

Frequently, small droplets or fragments of material will be left in the tip of the

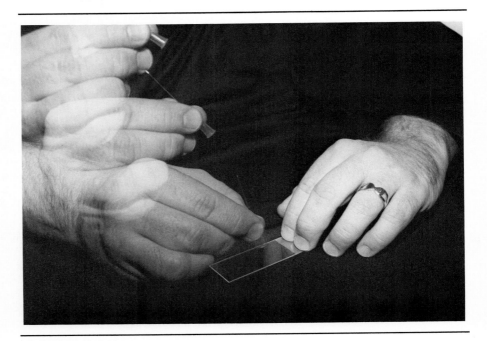

Figure 1.43.
*By holding the needle in this fashion and forcefully striking the open end of its hub against the glass slide, tissue particles lodged in the hub can be deposited on the slide for smearing.*

syringe, and tissue must be recovered from the syringe. We recover this in the following manner. The syringe without the needle is held as in Figure 1.15, and it is gently filled with air. The open end is placed on the glass slide and the plunger is rapidly, forcefully, and audibly pushed back to the empty position. This maneuver can be rapidly repeated several times so that all material can be recovered. It can then be collected and smeared, as described for tissue that was recovered from the needle hub. That is, small amounts can be handled with the two-step or modified two-step smearing techniques. If clotting occurs, a cell block should be prepared.

An alternative to this simple method involves rinsing of the syringe and needle with saline or fixative. We rarely use this method, as the material obtained requires concentration by centrifugation or filtration, with its attendant disadvantages. (Once again, the emphasis is on simple, rapid, and inexpensive means of specimen handling that can be accomplished at the bedside.)

After smears are prepared, some workers routinely rinse the needle and syringe with saline or fixative. This fluid is then centrifuged and examined for tumor cells. We prospectively studied 159 such needle-rinse specimens obtained at FNA of 152 patients. Aspiration sites included the breast (70), lymph nodes (30), lung (15), soft tissue (14), salivary glands (12), thyroid (12), liver (5), and a single branchial-cleft cyst. Malignancy was identified on smear material from 21 aspirates. In 16 of these (76%), the needle rinse material was also positive. No additional malignancies were detected by study of rinse material.[9]

We concluded that routine preparation and study of needle-rinse material contributes little to many FNA diagnoses. It is important to note, however, that in all cases, efforts were made to recover material from the syringe tip and the needle hub, as previously described. In the absence of such retrieval methods, needle-rinse material may be useful. Furthermore, because many malignancies will be represented in the rinse specimen, this method can be used to prepare additional slides if these are needed for special studies. This material can also be used to prepare histologic cell blocks, as previously discussed.

Although routine preparation and examination of slides from needle-rinse material may be unnecessary and inefficient, collecting this material at the bedside requires very little additional time or effort. Thus, some workers routinely rinse the needle and syringe at the time of FNA and then process this rinse-material specimen only in the minority of cases in which additional material is needed.

## ROUTINE AND RAPID STAINS

Unless intended for special studies or for cell-block embedding as a histologic specimen, the aspirated material can only be handled in two ways. Once a smear is prepared, it can be either fixed or dried. The choice between these alternatives should be made before the procedure is carried out because either one must be accomplished very rapidly once a smear has been prepared. Different stains are applied to these two types of slides, so that they initiate very different sequences of events in the laboratory.

Preferences vary among different microscopists. In general, fixed material is more often used in North America, and dried is more often used in Sweden. Often, a cytopathologist may prefer fixed slides for one kind of specimen and dried slides if other diagnostic possibilities are to be investigated. When someone other than the pathologist performs the aspiration, the laboratory should be consulted regarding the preferred handling of the slides.

The relative merits of the two methods are discussed in a subsequent subsection of this chapter. Because some processes are more easily diagnosed with one stain as opposed to another, and because surprises often occur in clinical medicine, we and others strive to prepare both dried and fixed slides in each case. It is often possible to split a single aspiration specimen into two or more slides, thus usually permitting preparation of a dried and a fixed slide from each aspiration specimen. We use this technique routinely, and in the majority of cases, both smears contain diagnostic material.

### Preparation of Smears Prior to Staining

Both methods of smear preparation are described next.

#### *Fixation of Smears*

Fixatives are applied to a smear as a spray or by immersion of the slide into a liquid. The liquid fixatives that have been used in cytopathology include 95 percent ethanol, 100 percent ethanol, sequential application of methanol and ethanol, 100 percent methanol, Saccomanno's fixative, combined methanol/ diethyl ether (Papanicolaou's fixative), acetone, 80 percent isopropyl alcohol, combined acetone/methanol, and Esposti's fixative (95% ethanol with 5% glacial acetic acid). The most commonly used is 95 percent ethanol; this inexpensive, readily available liquid provides excellent cytologic detail. Its only disadvantage is the need to store and transport unstained slides in a container of liquid and to have this fluid and these containers at hand in the clinic. We have found wet fixation in 95 percent ethanol highly suitable for immunocytochemistry (see subsequent discussion in this chapter).

The alternative to wet fixation is use of one of the commercially available spray fixatives. These generally consist of various mixtures containing either ethanol or isopropyl alcohol with polyethylene glycol. The latter leaves a coating on the slide after the alcohol has evaporated and is said to prevent cell shrinkage. Such sprayed slides are dry within a few seconds and are then suitable for storage, mailing, or immediate processing. These coating fixatives must first be removed with a 10-minute soak in 95 percent ethanol before staining is performed. If this step is hastened, poor-quality staining will result.

After this initial step, the staining of spray-fixed smears proceeds just as it would for wet-fixed smears. These commercial spray-fixative products can be purchased in small bottles with a finger pump, which are easily carried in the laboratory coat pocket by the roving practitioner of FNA. Many practitioners find these fixatives very convenient and easy to use.

Aerosol spray fixatives are also in use. Many gynecologists are accustomed to using hair spray to fix cervical smears. This is inexpensive, readily available, and works fairly well. Users of such methods must occasionally be reminded that aerosols expand rapidly when sprayed and thus are very cold. If the spray can is held closer to the smear surface than about 10 inches (25 cm), the cells will be rapidly frozen and severely damaged. The microscopic result very much resembles the air-drying artifact of fixed smears (discussed in the subsequent section) and frequently renders the material unsuitable for cytologic examination. Freedom from this freezing artifact makes the finger-pump type of spray fixative even more attractive.

Regardless of the fixative selected, it must be applied very quickly. Generally, good results are obtained only if it is applied within a few seconds of making a smear. Thus, the open container of ethanol or the bottle of spray must be placed next to the slides on which smears are to be made. When cells dry, they swell, and their sizes appear altered. Furthermore, the distinct details of nuclear structure are no longer seen. The effects of such drying artifact can be seen by comparing Figures 1.44 and 1.45. Even in well-fixed smears, some drying artifact may occur at the smear edges. Marked drying will render slides unsuitable for interpretation.

### Smear Drying

This simple procedure consists of rapidly and completely drying a smear before any stain is applied. This is usually accomplished by setting the smear aside. For optimal results, drying should occur quickly. The effects of slow drying on a

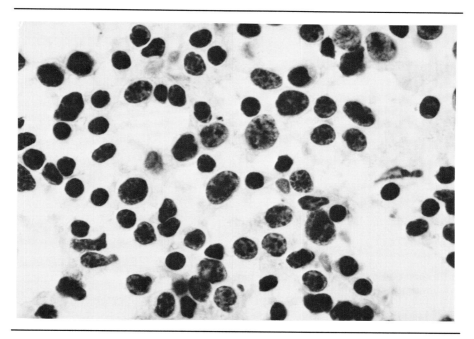

Figure 1.44.
*Fixed smear from a benign lymph node. This field shows lymphocytes with well-preserved rims of cytoplasm and sharp, distinct details of nuclear chromatin (Papanicolaou stain, magnification ×400 before a 34% reduction).*

fluid-rich smear were illustrated in Figure 1.35. Some go so far as to use a small battery-powered electric fan for rapid smear drying. We have not found this necessary, but we do sometimes hold a slide by the label and wave it gently in the air for a few seconds. This will hasten drying of a smear that has excess blood or fluid.

One advantage of the drying technique, when compared to wet or spray fixation, is that drying eliminates one technical step; drying smears basically consists of doing nothing. In this way, persons who perform occasional aspirations away from their usual clinic or hospital setting are relieved of the need to carry fixation materials. Also, dried smears (stained appropriately) are preferable to smears that have been badly or slowly fixed. The dried smears can be interpreted in the routine manner, while the poorly fixed ones are often difficult or impossible to interpret.

On occasion, we are consulted (usually at the last minute) by anxious clinicians about to perform one of their first aspirations and asked what is to be done with the slides. We usually suggest both air drying, which in most instances amounts to doing nothing but putting the slide aside, or spraying it "like a gynecologic smear." Ideally, both types of smears should be prepared.

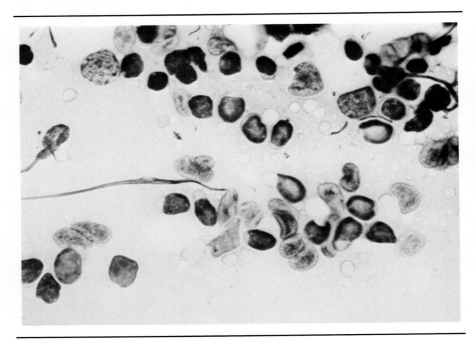

Figure 1.45.
*A slowly fixed (and thus dried) smear from the same case illustrated in Figure 1-44. The cells appear larger, are pale, and show very poor nuclear chromatin detail (Papanicolaou stain, magnification ×400 before a 34% reduction).*

## Routine Stains

Before we consider the use of particular stains for special studies, it is important to note that the actions taken by the laboratory depend on whether a slide has been fixed or dried.

### Stains Applied to Fixed Smears

Fixed material is usually stained by either the Papanicolaou or the hematoxylin and eosin (H&E) method. These stains are very much like those applied to paraffin-embedded histologic sections that form the basis of routine histopathology. Thus, they are immediately and intuitively attractive to those trained in surgical pathology.

Both employ one of the hematoxylins for staining of nuclei; this dye colors the nucleic acids a dark purplish-blue color. The counterstaining with eosin is designed to show cytoplasmic characteristics. The H&E stain can be performed very rapidly, as it is with frozen sections.

With the Papanicolaou stain, one hallmark is the use of orange G, which stains cytoplasmic keratin a bright orange color. This is very useful in identifying squamous differentiation. This fact forms part of the basis for its utility in searching for squamous-cell carcinoma of the uterine cervix and its precursors in gynecologic smears. It has been suggested that poor results will be obtained if slides are not kept completely wet during the Papanicolaou staining; nuclear details will not be rendered distinctly. Excessive draining between solutions should thus be avoided (Joseph Zajicek: personal communication to Dr. Löwhagen). The use of Papanicolaou stain in FNA is discussed subsequently herein, in regard to rapid staining techniques.

### Stains Applied to Air-Dried Smears

Any of several Romanowsky stains originally developed for application to blood and bone-marrow smears may be applied to air-dried smears. While numerous recipes exist, all are various combinations of methylene blue and its breakdown products (Azure A, B, or C) with eosin.[10] Most rely on methanol fixation. The most fundamental difference between these stains and those previously discussed is that they are applied to dried rather than to fixed smears. Cell drying results in cell swelling, so that cells tend to appear larger in Romanowsky preparations.

An important chemical characteristic is the ability of Romanowsky stains to react metachromatically with a variety of tissue components. This is a shifting of the dye's absorption spectrum in the presence of negatively charged entities, to give a reddish-purple color. Such reactions can be observed in nucleic acids (nuclear or nucleolar), various epithelial mucins, and extracellular matrix components. As illustrated at the end of this chapter, many of these substances are stained poorly or not at all with the Papanicolaou or H&E stains. Color Plates I through III show a case stained with H&E, Papanicolaou, and a Romanowsky stain, respectively.

## Rapid Staining Techniques

In many clinical situations, rapid results are desired. High-quality, rapid staining procedures are widely available and give excellent results. Many pathologists use an H&E stain adapted from the frozen section suite. These typically can be performed in 2 to 3 minutes.

### Rapid Papanicolaou Stains

Rapid Papanicolaou stains give results comparable to those obtained by longer methods and, depending on the recipe in use, can be completed in 3 to 7 minutes. Some manufacturers supply rapid-staining setups including all reagents. For example, the RAPID-CHROME™ kit from Shandon, Inc. (Pittsburgh, Pennsylvania) requires about 7 minutes. A method employed in our laboratory produces good-quality stains in about 3 minutes. The basis for such a method is mixing of the counterstains (eosin, light green, and orange G) to form a single staining step. This method is summarized in Table 1.5. In all such methods, liquid fixatives will be faster than spray fixatives because the latter require several minutes in 95 percent ethanol for complete removal.

When rapid Papanicolaou stains are performed outside the cytology laboratory (in the radiology suite, for example), xylene substitutes can be used. These often employ pleasant-smelling citrus terpenes and lack the irritating qualities of xylene. We have used Americlear (Fischer Scientific, Pittsburgh, Pennsylvania) with success.

Table 1.5
*Rapid Papanicolaou staining method, applied to wet fixed cytology smears*

|  | Reagent | Time |
|---|---|---|
| 1. | Tap water | 5 to 10 dips |
| 2. | Gill's hematoxylin* | 30 seconds to 1 minute |
| 3. | Tap water | 5 dips |
| 4. | Tap water | 10 seconds |
| 5. | Composite counterstain[†] | 30 seconds |
| 6. | Tap water | 10 dips |
| 7. | Tap water | 10 dips |
| 8. | 100% ethanol | 10 dips |
| 9. | 100% ethanol | 10 dips |
| 10. | Xylene or substitute | 5 dips |
| 11. | Xylene or substitute | 5 dips |
| 12. | Coverslip | |

*Reagents:* Commercial xylene substitutes may be used. See text for details.

*Gill's hematoxylin: Shandon, Inc. (Pittsburg, Pennsylvania).

†Composite counterstain: 50% EA-65 and 50% OG-6; both from Shandon, Inc. (Pittsburg, Pennsylvania).

## Rapid Romanowsky Stains

Rapid Romanowsky stains are also available. The ones we use are a modified Diff-Quik® stain[11] and a rapid May-Grünwald Giemsa (MGG) method developed at the Karolinska Hospital. The former involves alteration of the manufacturer's suggested staining times, to allow adequate fixation and staining of aspirated tissue fragments. The method is summarized in Table 1.6. Most of the Romanowsky-stained smears illustrated in this book were prepared with this method.

Table 1.6
*Modified Diff-Quik® stain for rapid Romanowsky staining of aspiration smears: Applied to air-dried smears*

|  | Reagent | Time |
|---|---|---|
| 1. | Absolute methanol | 2 minutes* |
| 2. | Solution I | 1 minute* |
| 3. | Solution II | 45 seconds† |
| 4. | Tap water | Rinse completely |
| 5. | Slide examination | |
|  | a.   Coverslip with water (temporary) | |
|  | b.   Examine without coverslip | |
|  | c.   Dry completely, immerse in xylene, and coverslip permanently | |

*Suggested minimum times.

†After initial staining, rinse the slide in tap water, blot semidry, and examine for staining quality. If additional staining is needed, place back in Solution II for 10 to 15 seconds. This restaining can be repeated as necessary and prevents overstaining. As the solutions age, the staining time in Solution II will lengthen.

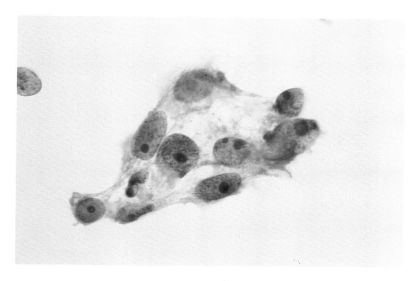

Color Plate I
*This breast-carcinoma smear has been stained with an H&E stain, just as a frozen section would be stained (enlarged 300%, × 312).*

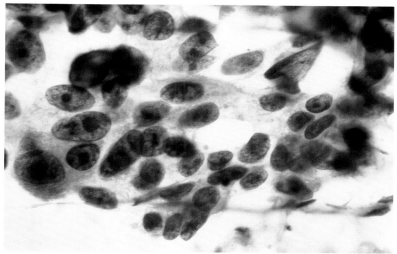

Color Plate II
*The same breast carcinoma shown in Color Plate I has been stained with a Papanicolaou stain (enlarged 300%, × 312).*

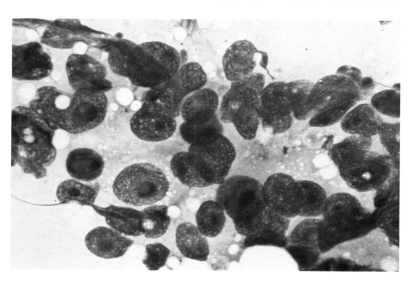

Color Plate III
*The breast carcinoma seen in Color Plates I and II is shown here with a Romanowsky stain (modified Diff- Quik® stain, enlarged 300%, × 312).*

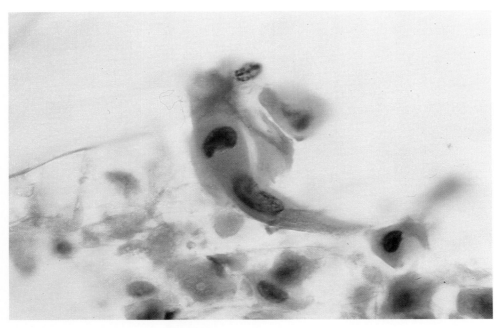

Color Plate IV
*This squamous-cell carcinoma of the lung shows keratinized malignant cells. These have brightly orangeophilic cytoplasm and very distinct cell borders (Papanicolaou stain, enlarged 375%, × 312).*

Color Plate V
*The same carcinoma shown in Color Plate IV is illustrated here with a Romanowsky stain. The cytoplasmic keratin is stained a deep blue color (modified Diff-Quik® stain, enlarged 375%, × 312).*

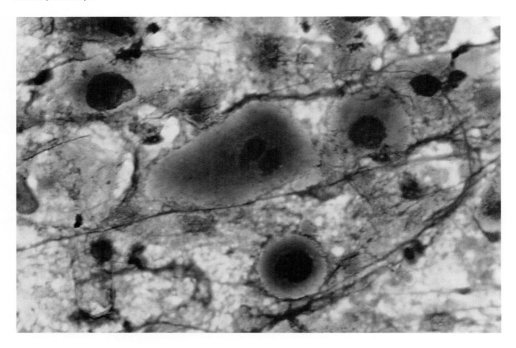

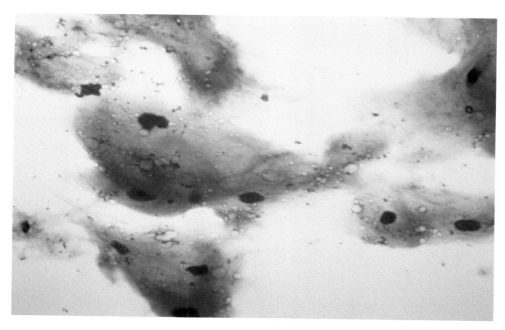

Color Plate VI
*This Romanowsky-stained smear from a mucinous carcinoma of the breast shows the extracellular mucin clearly as blue-staining wispy material surrounding the cellular elements. The tumor cell groups appear as round cell balls at this very low magnification (modified Diff-Quik® stain, enlarged 375%, × 31).*

Color Plate VII
*This alcohol-fixed, Papanicolaou-stained smear from the same case of mucinous breast carcinoma seen in Color Plate VI shows that with this stain, the extracellular mucin is nearly invisible. The tumor cells appear as round cell balls at this very low magnification (enlarged 375%, × 60).*

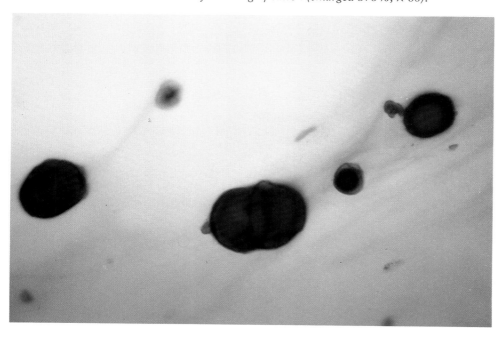

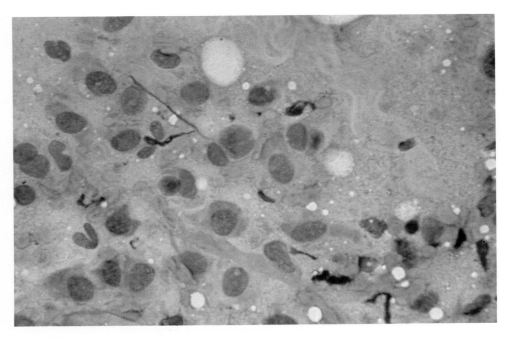

Color Plate VIII
*This Romanowsky-stained smear from a mucinous mixed tumor (pleomorphic adenoma) of the parotid gland shows distinct, red-staining droplets of cytoplasmic mucin (MGG stain, enlarged 375%, × 400).*


Color Plate IX
*This Romanowsky-stained benign prostatic epithelium contains large, irregularly shaped, metachromatic granules. These are evidence that a given group of cells is benign (modified Diff-Quik® stain, enlarged 375%, × 312).*

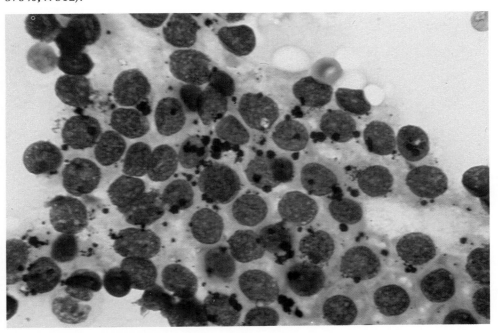

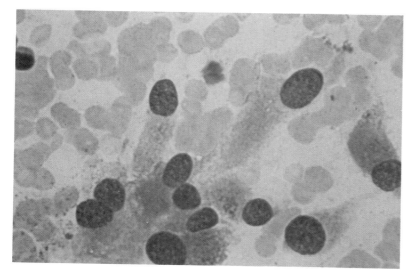

Color Plate X
*This medullary thyroid carcinoma shows fine, red, cytoplasmic granules. These are seen in approximately 20 percent of such cases (May-Grünwald Giemsa [MGG] stain, enlarged 300%, × 400).*

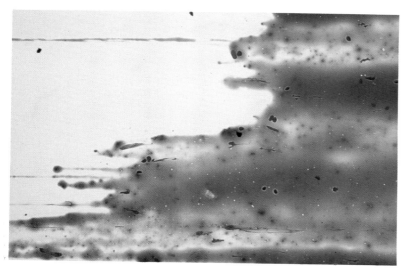

Color Plate XI
*This smear from a benign colloid nodule (nodular hyperplasia) of the thyroid shows abundant colloid. On this Romanowsky-stained preparation, it is deep purple (modified Diff-Quik® stain, enlarged 300%, × 312).*

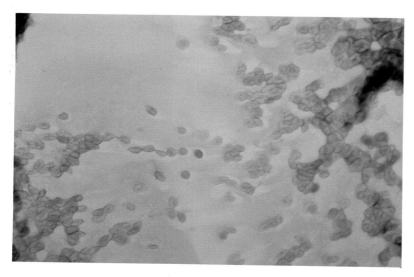

Color Plate XII
*The same case shown in Color Plate XI is here stained with the Papanicolaou method. The colloid is a pale pink color and is much less obvious (enlarged 300%, × 312).*

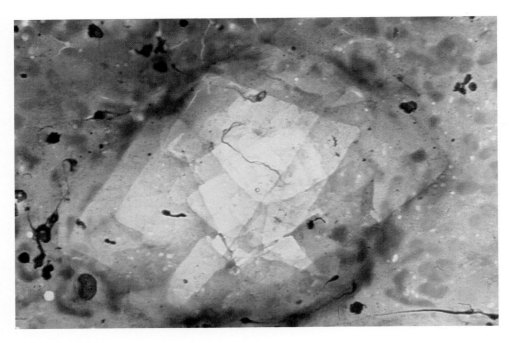

Color Plate XIII
*The apparent rectangular windowpanes seen in this thyroid colloid represent crystals that have been dissolved out during smear processing (modified Diff-Quik® stain, enlarged 375%, × 120).*

Color Plate XIV
*Papillary thyroid carcinoma (histologic section) showing intense hypereosinophilia of the colloid (H&E stain, enlarged 375%, × 120).*

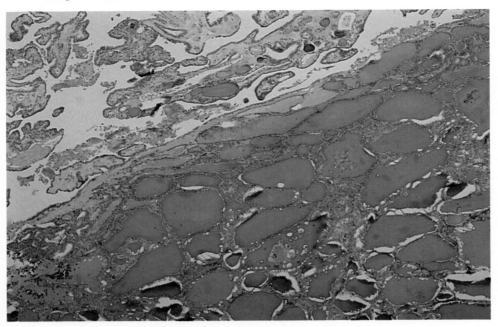

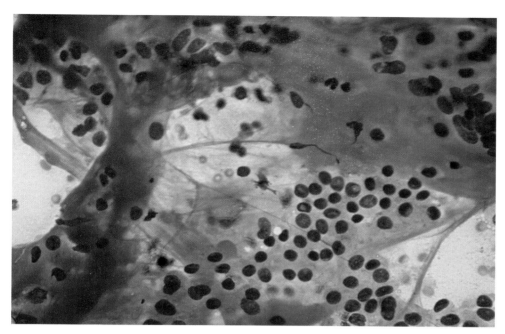

Color Plate XV
*Abnormal colloid from a case of papillary carcinoma of the thyroid. In contrast to the usual diffuse, carpetlike colloid illustrated in Color Plate XI, this shows a thick fibrillar or ropy appearance (modified Diff-Quik® stain, enlarged 375%, × 120).*

Color Plate XVI
*Smears from a benign mixed tumor of parotid gland origin show typical metachromatic, fibrillar matrix (modified Diff-Quik® stain, enlarged 375%, × 120).*

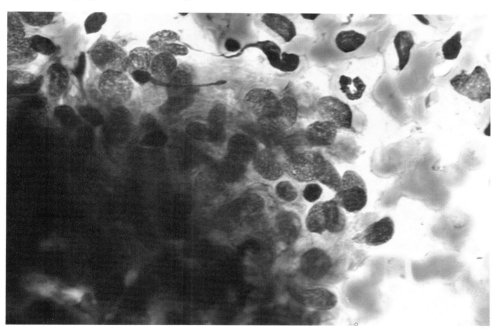

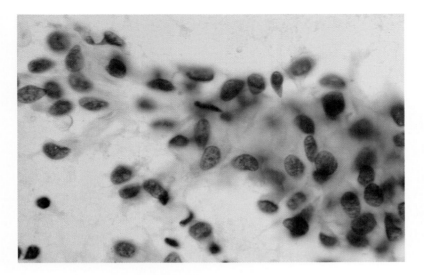

Color Plate XVII
*The same matrix is seen with the Papanicolaou stain (enlarged 300%, × 120). When present only in small quantity, however, this diagnostically important material is more easily identified in air-dried material such as that seen in Color Plate XVI.*

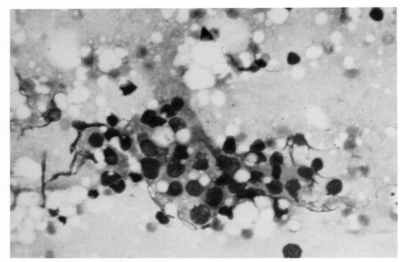

Color Plate XVIII
*This Romanowsky-stained smear from the breast of a lactating patient shows epithelial cells. Their being set in this characteristic blue-staining, frothy background is a very helpful clue to their true nature (modified Diff-Quik® stain, enlarged 300%, × 312).*

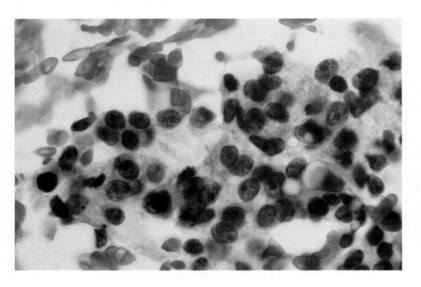

Color Plate XIX
*This Papanicolaou-stained smear from a lactating breast shows epithelial cells with enlarged, crowded nuclei and small nucleoli. Interpretation is made more difficult by the absence of the characteristic background seen in air-dried material (Color Plate XVIII) (enlarged 300%, × 400).*

The Karolinska Hospital rapid MGG stain is even simpler to apply. It requires only two staining steps and running water. It can be applied in 90 seconds, with excellent results. The method and reagents are summarized in Table 1.7. The staining can be allowed to continue as long as necessary because overstaining does not occur after saturation of the cells with pigment. Furthermore, prolonged fixation in methanol has no deleterious effect. Thus, if additional staining is needed after rapid evaluation (an uncommon problem), the slide can be added to the staining cart with the day's routine smears and processed again in the usual manner.

Overstaining does not occur with the Karolinska MGG method. In the Diff-Quik® method, however, cells left too long in Solution II will quickly darken and lose considerable microscopic detail. Thus, the Karolinska stain is rapid, simple, and virtually foolproof.

Installing a permanent coverslip on Romanowsky-stained slides in the conventional manner requires that the slides dry completely before immersion in the appropriate solvent (xylene or its substitutes). To avoid this delay, we often examine these smears before they have been coverslipped. Only at magnifications greater than 100x does this present a somewhat blurred image. Because low and intermediate magnifications are sufficient for diagnosis of most FNA specimens, many can be examined immediately (while still wet), without sacrifice of diagnostic accuracy.

If high-power viewing is needed, the slide can be moistened with tap water, and a coverslip can be applied immediately, with water as a mounting medium. The resulting image is always very clear. This water-mounting method permits rapid, high-quality examination (for example, in the radiology suite), without the need to transport and handle the organic solvents and sticky mounting media used for permanent coverslip application. After initial rapid examination, the coverslip is removed, and the slide should be dried thoroughly before application of a permanent coverslip. This final step is performed at the leisure of laboratory personnel, removed from the pressure to make a rapid diagnosis. Examination of the smear before permanent mounting by either of these methods can contribute to rapid diagnosis when this is needed.

Table 1.7
*Karolinska Hospital method for rapid May-Grünwold Giemsa stain*

|   | Reagent | Time |
|---|---|---|
| 1. | Absolute methanol | 30 seconds |
| 2. | Working Giemsa stain* | 1 minute |
| 3. | Rinse | Briefly in running tap water |

*One part Giemsa stock solution, diluted with 4 parts tap water. (Working solution should be changed daily.) Giemsa stock solution (stable at room temperature in amber glass):

| | |
|---|---|
| Azur II–eosin | 0.60 gm |
| Azur II | 0.16 gm |
| Glycerol | 50.00 gm |
| Methanol | to 100.00 gm total |

Stains are obtained from Merck (Damstadt, FDR): (a) Azur II—Catalog Number 9211; (b) Azure II–eosin—Catalog Number 9203 (Giemsa-Azur-Eosin-Methyleneblau für de Mikroscopi)

One rapid method of Romanowsky staining that we have found unacceptable is the use of slide-staining machines that are often found in large-volume routine hematology laboratories. These stains are often of poor quality. Furthermore, their quality varies greatly from slide to slide.

Instead, these aforementioned rapid Romanowsky stains (modified Diff-Quik® or Karolinska MGG) can be applied in minutes, using two or three stain containers. The ability to apply these stains is easily acquired and will greatly facilitate rapid examination of FNA material. We strongly suggest that FNA cytopathologists add this basic skill to their repertoire, thus becoming free from the need always to have a laboratory assistant available. This is similar to the freedom and rapidity that comes with being able to make smears or other preparations from aspirated material. After all, these stains are simpler to apply than the Gram stains that medical students still perform. In this way, important clinical problems can literally be solved within a few minutes at minimum cost.

## Preparation of Slides for Immunocytochemical Stains

As indicated previously, the majority of FNA specimens can be readily interpreted using routine stains applied to smears made at the bedside. These methods are inexpensive and give results quickly. A small number of cases, however, will require application of more advanced techniques. Many of these methods involve details of technique and controls that are only available in referral laboratories, where more than occasional cases require such studies. Cases of such difficulty or complexity may also require consultation with expert diagnosticians. Awareness of the available methods and basic understanding of specimen handling requirements will help ensure that proper material is available or can be obtained as needed.

Classification of malignant neoplasms has been greatly facilitated by modern immunocytochemical (ICC) methods. Tissue or cellular components are first bound by a specific primary antibody. These sites of binding are then revealed when one of a variety of labeling schemes is applied. Labeling employs enzyme-linked secondary antibodies that react with chromogen molecules to give an insoluble, colored reaction product. Microscopically visualized chromogen deposition then reveals the location of the tissue component of interest. Tumor immunophenotyping based on application of antibody panels has considerable utility in classifying difficult cases.

These methods are readily adapted to cytologic material, including that obtained by FNA. An important issue is optimum specimen preparation for maximum antigen preservation and minimum background nonspecific staining. Most ICC stains cannot be applied to routine air-dried smears. This is especially true if antibodies are applied over an existing Romanowsky stain. On the other hand, air-dried smears that are fixed briefly in cold (4°C) acetone and stored at −70°C can be stained for a wide variety of tissue elements.

Many ICC stains can be applied to fixed smears. These can be either separate slides prepared specifically for this purpose or slides previously stained by the method of Papanicolaou. We occasionally repeat an aspiration specifically to prepare slides or a cell block for ICC.

Whether new or previously stained, slides for ICC should be wet fixed by immediate immersion in 95 percent ethanol. Spray fixatives should not be used, as poor staining will result. This method of wet fixation can be simplified as follows: Fix the slides in 95 percent ethanol for 30 minutes, and then remove them from the liquid and allow them to dry. They can be transported or stored for 1 or 2 days in a form suitable for ICC. This avoids the decrease in antigenicity that follows long periods of exposure to fixatives.

An excellent way of preparing aspirated material for ICC is the embedded cell block discussed earlier. Multiple sections can be prepared for application of several primary antibodies. Most of the staining methods in common use were developed for formalin-fixed, paraffin-embedded tissue sections and are efficiently transferred to cytology cell blocks.

Immunostaining of cell-surface markers for phenotypic analysis of lymphoproliferative disorders requires special preparation of aspirated cells. This is discussed briefly in Chapter 2 when lymph node FNA is considered. These and other methods for application and interpretation of ICC stains to FNA specimens have recently been reviewed extensively.[12]

## Comparison of Fixed (Papanicolaou-Stained) and Dried (Romanowsky-Stained) Cytologic Material

Stains applied to fixed material are intuitively appealing to histopathologists. Only through extensive exposure can understanding and an intuitive grasp of a new method be acquired. We suggest (and others agree) that air-dried material has many advantages and deserves careful consideration by those using only the H&E or Papanicolaou methods. The senior author (TL) has for years taught FNA courses to groups of pathologists in many parts of the world. In these courses, he intentionally avoids showing fixed material during the initial phase of exposure to MGG-stained FNA smears. After 2 or 3 days of intensive exposure to the MGG stain, many not only see its utility, but also come to like and even prefer this method. Those who look at an occasional slide that was also stained by a Romanowsky method are not likely to acquire this skill.

Because highly reliable diagnosis occurs in some laboratories using mostly fixed smears and in other laboratories using mostly dried slides, much of the difference amounts to personal preference based on training and experience. Nonetheless, differences do exist; some of these are useful in certain circumstances, are summarized in Table 1.8.

### Cell Size

One fundamental difference between the two methods is that of apparent cell size. Air drying results in an increase in cell size due to apparent swelling. It has been shown that much of this change is actually due to flattening of the cells as drying occurs. This change has been described as an enlargement of nuclear areas.[13] The increase in apparent nuclear area is approximately 20 percent.[14,15] It is simple to show that this translates into a dried-cell nuclear diameter of 110 percent of the fixed-cell nuclear diameter. Furthermore, Schulte[15] found that the coefficient of variation in measured nuclear size was less with dried than with

Table 1.8
*Comparison of Papanicolaou and Romanowsky stains, as applied to aspiration cytology*

| Cytologic Finding | Papanicolaou Stain | Romanowsky Stain |
|---|:---:|:---:|
| Nuclear detail | + | |
| Cytoplasmic keratin | + | |
| Cytoplasmic mucin | | + |
| Cytoplasmic granules* | | + |
| Extracellular mucin | | + |
| Thyroid colloid | | + |
| Extracellular matrix material† | | + |
| Close resemblance of cells from malignant lymphoma or other hematopoietic processes to those seen in standard hematologic preparations | | + |

*Seen in benign prostatic epithelium, in many breast carcinomas, and in approximately 20% of medullary thyroid carcinomas.

†Cartilage, osteoid, mesenchymal myxoid material, and the characteristic chondroid matrix of parotid pleomorphic adenoma.

fixed material. Thus, it seems that dried slides may be more suitable for those wishing to perform morphometric studies or for those seeking to derive prognostic information from nuclear measurements as an expression of tumor grade.[16–21]

### Nuclear Detail

The most commonly cited advantage of fixed material is the exquisite nuclear detail available with this method. Color Plates I and II show crisp details of nuclear morphology, including shape, membrane contours, nuclear membrane thickness, chromatin clumping pattern, and chromatin distribution. In traditional exfoliative cytology, it is precisely these details of nuclear morphology that form the basis for deciding that the cells in question originated in a malignant process. On the other hand, as illustrated in Color Plate III, chromatin details are less clear in air-dried material. This illustrates why most pathologists still prefer to apply Papanicolaou staining to fixed smears in the assessment of exfoliated cells in sputum, urine, cervical scrapings and brushings, or washing of the gastrointestinal or respiratory tracts. We certainly agree with this approach to exfoliated cells.

FNA, however, often gives a much larger number of tumor cells than are present in exfoliated material and frequently yields tissue fragments as well. These tissue particles represent small biopsies and frequently reveal information about tumor architecture, stromal elements, extracellular tissue components, and the relations of tumor cells to one another. In this way, tissue particles and smear cellularity are the cytologists' equivalent of the histopathologists' concept of tissue architecture. Analysis of fine details of nuclear chromatin is replaced by other significant features, including smear pattern, cellularity, tissue fragment analysis, cell or nuclear size, degree of nuclear staining, and cell variability. This is reflected by the fact that many FNA specimens are most effectively examined at a low or intermediate magnification, just as histologic sections are studied.

This use of low or medium magnification for aspirated material is in contrast with the frequent need to use high magnification for detailed study of small numbers of cells in exfoliative cytology. Of course, exceptions occur. FNA specimens of low cellularity occasionally are encountered, sometimes for technical reasons. For example, the pathologic characteristics of some tumors simply preclude a richly cellular aspiration. This is so characteristic of some neoplasms, such as lobular carcinoma of the breast or purely intraductal breast carcinoma (as opposed to infiltrating ductal carcinoma), that it constitutes one of the criteria for diagnosis. In such cases, the morphology of individual tumor cells must be considered in detail. When this occurs, the examiner will compare them to a mental image gained from more cellular examples of the same entity or from similar cases encountered in the past. ("The cells are few in number, but they appear typical of breast carcinoma.") In such instances, the situation alluded to earlier obtains; the preferred stain is the one most familiar to the individual who is examining the smears. Some of the contrasts between FNA and exfoliative cytology are summarized in Table 1.9.

## Cytoplasmic Differentiation

The Papanicolaou stain was in part devised to reveal keratin as an indicator of squamous differentiation. Considering the common occurrence of squamous-cell carcinomas and their metastases, this is an important use of this stain. The cytoplasmic keratin in squamous-cell carcinomas avidly binds the orange G cytoplasmic counterstain of the Papanicolaou formulations, as illustrated in Color Plate IV. The same case stained by the modified Diff-Quik® method shows deep blue staining of the keratin (Color Plate V). The nuclei of these cells are large, densely hyperchromatic, irregularly shaped, and often lack nucleoli. While these features are seen with either stain, the cytoplasmic differentiation as manifested by keratin production is more vivid in the fixed material (Papanicolaou stain). Aspirations from such tumors often have diagnostic cells scattered through large areas of blood, necrotic debris, and inflammatory cells. It is very helpful to have the bright-orange tumor cells stand out so clearly. On the other hand, these cases are rare in commonly aspirated sites such as the breast and thyroid, so that this is not a reason to employ the Papanicolaou stain in all FNA material.

Table 1.9
*Differences in aspiration cytology and exfoliative cytology*

|  | Aspiration Cytology | Exfoliative Cytology |
|---|---|---|
| **Smear findings** | | |
| High cellularity | Common | Uncommon |
| Tissue fragments | Common | Uncommon |
| **Smear examination** | | |
| Pattern | Very important | Less important |
| Nuclear features | Less important | Very important |
| Use of high magnification | Occasionally | Frequently |

A variety of cytoplasmic granules and vacuoles have been described and are easily demonstrated using air-dried smears. After all, these subtle indicators of cytoplasmic differentiation are of paramount importance in the hematologic material for which these stains were initially developed. Many of these are visualized poorly or not at all in fixed material. An important example is the large, irregularly shaped, metachromatic granules seen in benign prostatic epithelium (Color Plate VI). These are presumed to be lysosomal in nature and would be very unusual in a group of malignant cells. Another example is the fine red cytoplasmic granulation seen in 20 percent of medullary thyroid carcinomas (Color Plate VII).

### Extracellular Materials

We and others[22,23] have noted that extracellular mucin is much more easily identified in air-dried smears. If present in small quantities, it may be nearly invisible on fixed preparations. The appearance of extracellular mucin from a mucinous carcinoma of the breast is shown with both stains in Color Plates VIII and IX. Small droplets of intracellular mucin are well shown by the Romanowsky stain because they may be metachromatic (Color Plate X).

In thyroid cytology, the presence, quantity, and quality of colloid is of diagnostic significance. When abundant and free of blood, colloid can be identified grossly as a clear oily-appearing substance as the smear is prepared. If mixed with cyst fluid or blood, its presence may not be grossly appreciated. Microscopically, it is much more readily apparent in Romanowsky-stained than in Papanicolaou-stained smears (cf. Color Plates XI and XII).

When lesions of the thyroid or other organs are partially cystic, they often contain crystals. These will dissolve away in the organic solvents used for either type of stain. In the dried material, a background of deeply stained colloid will show clear spaces or apparent windowpanes that represent the negative image of the crystals (Color Plate XIII). While of no great diagnostic utility, these are often very beautiful but will usually not be seen in Papanicolaou-stained smears.

One more aspect of thyroid colloid deserves comment. The colloid in papillary carcinoma differs from that of the normal gland in some as-yet biochemically uncharacterized way. Histologically, this is reflected in its hypereosinophilia. As shown in Color Plate XIV, such colloid is often intensely red. When seen in smears, it also differs from that illustrated in Color Plate XI. It tends to be either fibrillar and ropy or to form small, spherical, densely staining eosinophilic droplets (Color Plate XV). This special colloid, though usually not abundant, is a feature supporting the diagnosis of papillary carcinoma. It is very difficult to detect on a fixed, Papanicolaou-stained preparation.

A variety of extracellular materials other than colloid and the epithelial mucins are of diagnostic importance. The first that we consider here is the *chondroid matrix*, which is typical of the benign mixed tumor (pleomorphic adenoma) of salivary glands. This common tumor accounts for as much as 80 percent of salivary-gland neoplasms studied by FNA. While highly diverse (hence, the designation *pleomorphic*), the underlying themes of its histopathology are epithelial ductlike structures and myoepithelial cells. The latter are thought to be responsible for elaboration of the extracellular matrix. This material is highly characteristic, and even when present only in small

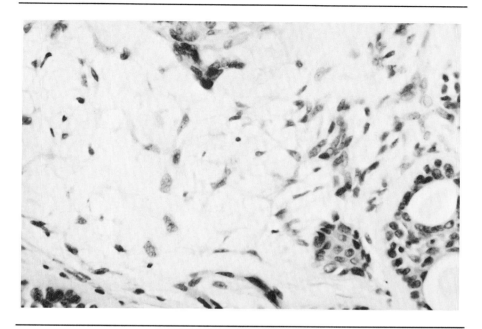

Figure 1.46.
*This histologically typical benign mixed tumor (pleomorphic adenoma) of the parotid gland consists of ducts and spindled myoepithelial cells, set in abundant, pale chondroid matrix of their own elaboration (H&E stain, magnification ×120 before a 28% reduction).*

quantities, it is a helpful diagnostic finding. The histology of a typical example is shown in Figure 1.46.

This myoepithelial-cell material is also helpful in cytologic smears. When abundant, it is readily recognized in either stain. It appears somewhat fibrillar in both, but with the Romanowsky stain, it is bright red. When it is present in only small amounts, it is much more easily identified and characterized in dried material. Thus, we find highly cellular (matrix deficient) examples of mixed tumor much easier to confidently diagnose when air-dried smears are available (Color Plates XVI and XVII).

Another common situation is aspiration of the breast during pregnancy or lactation. The cytologic changes of intense metabolic activity in these settings is a well-known cause of false-positive diagnoses of malignancy. The cytology during pregnancy or lactation is actually rather characteristic, consisting of nuclear enlargement, mostly round nuclei, prominent nucleoli, and a tendency of the cells to be arranged in small acinar groups. Their abundant cytoplasm is fragile, so that many of the cells appear as large, round, naked nuclei. The air-dried smear also shows a characteristic background. The secretory material and cytoplasmic fragments are present in the smear background as a blue staining, frothy, or vacuolated material (Color Plate XVIII). We find this very helpful in the secure identification of lactational or secretory changes. This background is much less apparent in fixed smears (Color Plate XIX).

In a variety of conditions, extracellular myxoid matrix materials can be obtained by aspiration. (These are connective-tissue-type ground substances rather than the extracellular epithelial mucins previously described.) These can be seen in conditions as diverse as *nodular fasciitis* (a benign, often self-limited, nonrecurring proliferation of myofibroblasts), *malignant fibrous histiocytoma* (a common type of soft tissue sarcoma), and chordoma. So while not diagnostically specific, they form a helpful part of the cytologic picture in many soft-tissue masses. Such materials are much more easily identified in Romanowsky-stained preparations in which they are red; they may be nearly invisible on fixed smears.

### Hematopoietic Processes

Malignant lymphomas, leukemias, and reactive processes are common and may pose formidable diagnostic problems. These may be addressed with a variety of special techniques, which are briefly discussed when lymph-node aspiration is considered in Chapter 2. The first step remains careful evaluation of high-quality smears.

Those with experience in hematopathology will find air-dried, Romanowsky-stained material very comparable to the bone marrow and blood smears that they are accustomed to studying. This is a very important use of air-dried specimens, especially in lymph-node FNA.

The foregoing discussion and examples are intended to suggest ways in which we have found one stain or the other to be preferable in different types of cases. Such a catalog could be extended indefinitely and would reflect the biases of its authors. Our point is that the method to be preferred depends on the differential diagnostic considerations at hand, as well as the preference and experience of the cytopathologist. Thus, it is advisable to collect both air-dried and fixed material whenever feasible. Clinicians who obtain their own specimens should consult the laboratory frequently.

# REFERENCES

1. Martin HE, Ellis EB: Biopsy by needle puncture and aspiration. Ann Surg 1930;92: 169–181.
2. Franzen S, Giertz G, Zajicek J: Cytological diagnosis of prostatic tumors by transrectal aspiration biopsy: A preliminary report. Brit J Urol 1960;32:193–201.
3. Shune D: Transbronchial needle aspiration: Current status. Mayo Clin Proc 1989;64:251–254.
4. Nordenskjold B, Löwhagen T, Westerberg H, Zajicek J: $^3$H- thymidine incorporation into mammary carcinoma cells obtained by needle aspiration before and during therapy. Acta Cytol 1976;20:137–143.
5. Furnival CM, Hughes HE, Hocking MA, et al.: Aspiration cytology in breast cancer: Its relevance to diagnosis. Lancet 1975;2:446– 448.
6. Zajdela A, deMaüblanc MT, Schlienger P, Hage C: Cytologic diagnosis of periorbital palpable tumors using fine-needle sampling without aspiration. Diagn Cytopathol 1986;2:17–20.
7. Ciatto S, Catania S, Bravetti P, et al.: Fine needle cytology of the breast: A controlled study of aspiration versus nonaspiration. Diagn Cytopathol 1991;7:125–127.

8. Kung ITM, Chan S-K, Fung K-H: Fine-needle aspiration in hepatocellular carcinoma: Combined clinical, cytologic and histologic approach. Cancer 1991;67: 673–680.

9. Henry-Stanley MJ, Stanley MW: Processing of needle rinse material from fine needle aspirations rarely detects malignancy not seen in smears. Diagn Cytopathol: In press.

10. Wittekind DH, Gehring T: On the nature of Romanowsky-Giemsa staining and the Romanowsky–Giemsa effect: I. Model experiments on the specificity of Azure B-eosin Y stain as compared with other thiazine dye–eosin Y combinations. Histochemical J 1985;17:263–289.

11. Henry MJ, Burton LG, Stanley MW, Horwitz CA: Application of a modified Diff-Quik® stain to fine needle aspiration smears: Rapid staining with improved cytologic detail. Acta Cytol 1989;31:954–955.

12. Yazdi HM, Dardick I: Guides to clinical aspiration biopsy: Diagnostic immunocytochemistry and electron microscopy. New York: Igaku-Shoin, 1992.

13. Schulte E: Air drying as a preparatory factor in cytology. Diagn Cytopathol 1986;2:160–167.

14. Dziura DR, Bonfiglio TA: Needle cytology of the breast: A quantitative study of the cells of benign and malignant ductal neoplasia. Acta Cytol 1979;23:332–334.

15. Schulte E, Wittekind C: The influence of the wet-fixed Papanicolaou and the air-dried Giemsa techniques on nuclear parameters in breast cancer cytology: A cytomorphometric study. Diagn Cytopathol 1987;3:256–261.

16. Wallgren A, Zajicek J: The prognostic value of aspiration biopsy smear in mammary carcinoma. Acta Cytol 1976;20:479–485.

17. Zajdela A, De LaRiva LS, Ghossein NA: The relation of prognosis to the nuclear diameter of breast cancer cells obtained by cytologic aspiration. Acta Cytol 1979;23:75–80.

18. Cornelisse CJ, De Koning HR, Arentz PW, et al.: Quantitative analysis of the nuclear area variation in benign and malignant breast cytology specimens. Acta Cytol 1981;3:128–134.

19. Baak JPA, Kurver PHJ, Snoo-Nieuwlaat AJE, et al.: Prognostic indicators in breast cancer-morphometric methods. Histopathology 1982;6:327–339.

20. Fossa SD, Marton PF, Knudsen OS, et al.: Nuclear Feulgen DNA content and nuclear size in human breast carcinoma. Hum Pathol 1982;13:626–630.

21. Baak JPA, Van Dop H, Kurver PHJ, et al.: The value of morphometry to classic prognosticators in breast cancer. 1985;56:374–382.

22. Stanley MW, Tani EM, Skoog L: Mucinous breast carcinoma and mixed mucinous-infiltrating ductal carcinoma: A comparative cytologic study. Diagn Cytopathol 1989;5:134–138.

23. Frable WJ: Thin-needle aspiration biopsy. Philadelphia: Saunders, 1983:51–53.

# The Patient: Clinical Techniques and Results Reporting

**2**

## WHO SHOULD PERFORM FINE-NEEDLE ASPIRATIONS?

Clearly, there is no single best answer to this question. The primary responsibility for obtaining specimens by aspiration rests with different types of individuals in different institutions. The two existing systems of designating role assignments were mentioned in Chapter 1 and are implemented along largely geographical lines. In Sweden, a single individual often has the responsibility to see the patient, perform the aspiration, prepare the material obtained, examine the smears at the microscope and report the diagnosis. In North America, on the other hand, it is customary for different persons to see the patient and to perform the microscopy. In either system, the physician or physicians involved will frequently need to consult their colleagues in the radiology suite or in the microbiology laboratory.

The primary argument in favor of the North American style of separating these functions is that each physician is performing a limited role in which he or she has considerable expertise. Thus, the surgeon brings experience to the physical examination of mass lesions and to the performance of procedures directed at such lesions. These individuals are indeed very qualified to skillfully implement FNA. However, as illustrated in Chapter 1, we feel strongly that good results will depend on their having received training in aspiration and on having made provisions for proper handling of aspirated material by suitably schooled personnel.

When the clinician involved is not a surgeon but is a general internist, a gynecologist, or a general practitioner, the degree of expertise brought to the aspiration may be considerably less. Furthermore, these physicians may deal with patients in need of FNA only occasionally and thus may receive little ongoing practice in the method. It has been shown that those performing aspirations on an occasional basis do not obtain the excellent results possible with this technique. Others support our contention that aspirations must be performed frequently if skills adequate to sample small lesions are to be developed and maintained.[1,2]

Any physician can refer a patient for FNA, just as for a chest x-ray or other test. The method should be regarded as a first-line approach to the palpable mass (much as a chest radiograph, for example, would be for a chronic cough). FNA is thus an element of primary care. Many benign lesions will not require referral to a surgeon or other specialist. Those that do require referral will then be sent for the most appropriate type of care.

We suggest that most aspiration procedures be performed by an individual who does them often and who is experienced in the method. Precedent for this approach certainly exists for other clinical procedures, including venipuncture, electrocardiography, and endotracheal tube placement. In many centers, highly skilled teams, consisting of a few individuals, perform these procedures wherever needed. In this way, optimum results are consistently obtained, and patients receive the most rapid, skilled, atraumatic, and effective care during technical procedures.

There is ample support in the literature for the concept that the best results are obtained with the Swedish model.[3–7] The foregoing discussion suggests that the need for training, experience, and constant practice in the method is one reason for this. Hall et al. studied samples from 795 patients aspirated for evaluation of thyroid nodules. They found that inadequate aspirations were obtained in 32.4 percent of cases by community clinicians, in 15 percent of cases by medical-center clinicians, and in only 6.4 percent of cases aspirated by a cytopathologist.[7]

Other contributing factors to expert use of FNA include the immediate recognition of a correlation between the clinical impression of a mass and the gross appearance of the aspirated material. Many inadequate specimens can be recognized at once and the aspiration repeated immediately if the individual performing the procedure brings to the bedside expectations about the nature of the specimen to be produced. The constant review of specimens at the microscope, in concert with clinical examination of patients, is the only way to build this type of experience.

Furthermore, specimens can be accurately triaged by a cytopathologist at the time of the aspiration, based on differential diagnostic considerations, so that special studies will be available on a timely basis, without the need for frequent repeat aspirations. This takes advantage of the pathologist's special knowledge of laboratory methods for approaching a given diagnostic problem. As outlined in Chapter 1, either air-dried or fixed material may be strongly preferred by the microscopist, depending on the diagnostic considerations at hand. If the person who will be examining the material prepares the slides, either type of smear can be emphasized from the outset. Cell blocks can also be prepared, as needed.

Some feel that a surgeon or other qualified clinician should obtain the specimen because of expertise in physical examination and in the assessment of masses. When a pathologist performs aspirations, he or she will usually review the cytologic material within a few minutes to a few hours. What better way could there possibly be to learn the nature of masses felt through the skin? No other physician has such complete and immediate feedback. The pathologist who performs several aspirations a day is probably the most skilled assessor of lumps and bumps who could possibly be trained.

The reasons why we believe that the Swedish model works best are summarized in Table 2.1.

The case studies in Chapter 3 highlight some examples of the cytopathologist working as a vital member of a clinical team. Although the attending clinician oversees and coordinates patient care, an experienced, skilled cytopathologist can contribute rapid, acute diagnoses of mass lesions. Rather than usurping the clinician's authority, this approach increases his or her effectiveness by ensuring the best possible nonsurgical diagnosis of these lesions. The patient is thus approached by a team of physicians; each contributes to high-quality care. All information is ultimately synthesized by the attending clinician.

Thus far, we have considered who should perform the clinical procedure of FNA. It seems appropriate to reflect for a moment on who should interpret the material at the microscope. As this method gains acceptance, and as it intrudes on many facets of the medical literature, the demand for pathologists to interpret smears brought by clinicians is increasing rapidly. While a detailed description of the cytopathology of any body site is beyond the scope of this book, we agree with Tao et al. that "the so-called 'cytologic criteria of malignancy' as generally described in Pathology and Cytology books are not applicable on many occasions."[8]

We examined this issue from another perspective in Chapter 1, when we suggested that smear cellularity and tissue-particle morphology are often more

Table 2.1

*Suggested reasons why centralized performance of aspirations by a cytopathologist is the best way to ensure a high-quality FNA service*

1. Frequent performance of aspirations ensures the greatest possible technical expertise.

2. Immediate feedback by rapid microscopic diagnosis makes a busy cytopathologist the most skilled clinical assessor of palpable mass lesions.

3. Gross inspection of smears at the time of the procedure, with their expected microscopic appearance in mind, allows the cytopathologist to recognize and immediately repeat many inadequate aspirations.

4. The cytopathologist can emphasize either dried or fixed smears, as well as cell-block preparations at the time of the procedure, so that the specimen is tailored to the important differential diagnostic possibilities.

5. The specimen can be allocated for special studies, based on the pathologist's special knowledge of the laboratory methods for approaching a particular set of diagnoses.

6. Optimal integration of clinical, radiographic, and cytologic findings is achieved when a single individual reviews and correlates all diagnostic modalities.

7. The patient's history is often learned much more accurately and completely by talking to the patient than by depending on data provided by busy clinicians.

important to the diagnosis of FNA material than are the fine details of nuclear morphology that make up much of these "cytologic criteria of malignancy." Thus, FNA is not just an extension of traditional exfoliative cytology but in many instances represents a new type of material. Furthermore, the criteria for diagnosis, though more a reflection of surgical pathology than of exfoliative cytology, cannot be fully deduced or extrapolated from histopathology. For these reasons, special training is required if accurate interpretation is to result. Hajdu and Melamed state the issue clearly when they write, "unprepared pathologists should not yield to the pressures of making diagnoses. Under the medicolegal system in the United States, which is fundamentally different from that of many other countries, there is very little room for error in diagnosis."[9]

FNA thus joins the ranks of many modern techniques in which one cannot dabble and expect success.

## FUNDAMENTAL RULES FOR APPLYING ASPIRATION CYTOLOGY

In their essay on the limitations of FNA, Hajdu and Melamed outline the ground rules for clinical application of this method.[9] Many of these were clearly defined in early descriptions of the technique by Martin and Ellis, by Stewart, and by Soderstrom[10–12] and are summarized in Table 2.2.

First, aspiration is always directed at a target lesion. This can either be a palpable mass or a tumor localized radiographically. FNA is not a screening test used to search for possible malignancy, even in a high-risk population.

The next two of the three rules are really no different from the bases on which all biopsy pathology is practiced. Rule 2: A reasonable interpretation is possible only when the cytologic findings are placed in a clinical context. The minimum details needed are the age and sex of the patient, as well as the exact site of the aspiration. As we discuss subsequently in this chapter, additional information is often available clinically. The texture noted when a mass is penetrated by the needle and the nature of the aspirated material further enhance definition of the clinical landscape.

The third, very important principle is that in a patient thought to have a malignancy, a negative report that does not provide a specific benign diagnosis leaves the clinical problem unsolved. The mass must be addressed either by repeat aspiration or by some other diagnostic maneuver. Only a specific benign diagnosis (such as an infection) that presents a reasonable alternative explanation for the clinical findings is acceptable.

Table 2.2
*Ground rules for application of FNA*

1. Aspiration should always be aimed at a target lesion.
2. A diagnosis can be made only within a known clinical context.
3. Negative reports may leave the clinical problem unsolved.

# TALKING WITH PATIENTS BEFORE THE ASPIRATION

## Face-to-Face Communication with the Patient

The patient comes to the procedure with a range of possible expectations. In Sweden, where aspiration is common, many have some familiarity with the method and thus know something about what to expect. In North America, there are still many to whom the idea is completely new. The patients often arrive at the clinic prepared for a complex, painful procedure, which they think is implied by the word *biopsy*. We have encountered patients subjected to self-imposed overnight fasting who are prone to fainting. We try to approach patients in a relaxed and friendly manner that will put them at ease. Linsk and Franzen draw on extensive experience in clinical FNA to offer many valuable suggestions regarding a kind and thoughtful approach to anxious patients.[13]

The medicolegal standard in North America demands that all patients be completely informed about medical procedures. This includes all pertinent information on the risks, benefits, and alternatives to a given procedure. The risks of aspiration are quite minimal. One must create a balance between discussing such extremely remote events as pneumothorax and making an effort to put the patient at ease for what is a rapid, simple, and extremely safe procedure.

## Patient Information Brochure

We often use a brochure to communicate much of this basic information to our patients. This is modeled on the brochure developed by John Abele (of Sacramento, California) and used for several years in his large FNA practice. This can be provided in the clinic waiting room or can be given to the patient by the referring physician when an appointment for aspiration is made. We often rehearse some of the basic information with the patient before the procedure. We are always careful to provide an opportunity for the patient to ask any questions that may come to mind. Our brochure provides the information in the form of commonly asked questions, such as those that follow.

### What Is FNA?

FNA is a quick, reliable, comfortable method of diagnosing lumps that can be felt by you or your doctor. It is simple, requiring an appointment of only 10 to 15 minutes. We want to answer any questions you may have about FNA.

### Is FNA New?

No. The technique was invented in America more than 60 years ago. It is used widely on both coasts of our country. Its most extensive development, however, has been in Sweden. The preparation and interpretation of aspiration material has been refined in the past several years.

### What Is the Purpose of FNA?

When a lump is detected, possible treatments range from doing nothing more than to observe it over time to surgically removing it. Many lumps do not need to be removed except to answer the question, "what is it?" Others are more serious and do warrant surgery. FNA is used to obtain small amounts of tissue from a lump. Once your physician knows what the lump represents, she or he may be able to safely and confidently tell you that surgery is unnecessary. If, on the other hand, you do need surgery, your doctor can approach this complex process with a diagnosis in hand and can fully inform you about your options in treatment.

### What Is the FNA Process Like?

First, we ask you about the lump. When did you first notice it? Is it tender? Has it changed in any way? Have you had an injury, infection, or medical treatment in the area? Next, we review any x-rays or other reports from your doctor. Finally, we answer any questions you may wish to ask.

The procedure begins by accurately measuring and locating the lump, by feeling it with the fingertips. In this way, we can tell your doctor exactly what was sampled. The actual aspiration is brief, lasting only a few seconds. From your point of view, it will be much like getting an immunization injection. We use the smallest possible needle to obtain a reliable sample. The size we use is actually one of the smallest needles made. The skin is cleansed with alcohol and the needle is inserted for about 5 to 10 seconds. A sterile gauze pad is then pressed on the area for a few minutes. Most lumps require two to four such samples to ensure complete results. Occasionally, one is sufficient.

After the aspiration, you may return to your normal activities. Please continue to take all prescribed medications as usual because the aspiration will not affect these.

### What Are the Complications of FNA?

Because the needle is very small, this technique is virtually free of complications. A small bruise or tenderness may occur at the aspiration site. This is mild, requires no special treatment, and disappears in a few days. Actual bleeding at the time of aspiration is usually limited to a few drops. Complications such as rapid swelling or infection are extraordinarily rare. Nonetheless, should any problem arise after the biopsy, please notify your doctor immediately.

### How Are FNA Results Obtained?

The physician who performs your aspiration will personally examine the sample with the microscope. This system has been very successful around the world. In this way, the information obtained by examining you and feeling the lump can be added to what is seen through the microscope and to the important observations you have made before coming to the clinic.

### When Will You Know the Results?

We telephone results to your doctor's office within a few hours. A written report is then sent to your doctor, by mail or by facsimile ("fax"). We feel that your own physician is best able to explain what the results mean for you and what (if anything) should be done next.

*What Are the Limitations of FNA?*

Our goal is to determine the cause of your lump. In the vast majority of cases, this goal is achieved. In a few instances, the possibilities are at least narrowed to two or three likely choices. In a small percentage of cases, the sample is too limited to be helpful. Whenever the specific cause remains uncertain, your doctor might recommend repeat FNA, a surgical biopsy, or other studies.

Despite careful performance of FNA, no medical test is 100 percent accurate. The chance of FNA failing to find a malignancy when one is present is 1 to 5 percent. Thus, neither you nor your physician should forget about a lump after FNA. Instead, you should both continue to watch for any change. Should enlargement occur, it is imperative that it be resampled, either by FNA or by surgical biopsy.

## Additional Communication

With this information in hand, the patient knows why the procedure is being performed, what its goals are, what limitations apply, what to expect from the procedure, what the complications might be, how to obtain results, and how to behave after the procedure. Actually, in many instances, neither the brochure nor a prolonged discussion will be needed at the time of aspiration. Some patients will have been adequately prepared by the referring physician.

Most physicians do not require a signed consent for aspiration, having likened it to venipuncture.[2] We do not hesitate to perform this procedure on patients who are unable to communicate or are seriously ill and unable to benefit from the information just presented. In such grave situations, we often try to calm the patient or family members with very brief mention of the small size of the needle, the rapidity of the procedure, and the extreme rarity of serious complications. This can be done quickly and is often very welcome and reassuring. Indeed, it is these seriously ill individuals who may benefit most from the rapid, accurate diagnoses provided by FNA.

## CLINICAL APPLICATION OF THE ASPIRATION PROCEDURE

The basic motions of the aspiration procedure and the options for handling the material obtained were described in Chapter 1. These should be mastered before the patient is approached with a needle. Thus, even from the beginning, the procedure can go smoothly and need not alarm the patient unnecessarily.

The entire process should include several steps in addition to the puncture event itself. Ideally, the process is nothing less than a synthesis of clinical, radiographic, laboratory, historical, tactile, and cytologic findings to form a diagnosis that is as accurate and complete as possible. The various components of this process are summarized in Table 2.3. Although cumbersome to describe verbally, the entire process usually requires about 10 minutes to complete. As previously mentioned, the needle is in the mass for approximately 5 to 10 seconds

Table 2.3
*Stepwise FNA procedure*

1. Question the patient or the referring physician about the history of the mass and other significant medical problems.
2. Review any relevant radiographs and laboratory studies, consulting specialists in these areas, as necessary.
3. Examine the area to be aspirated.
4. Mentally plan the aspiration, with respect to stabilization of the mass, needle size, and number of punctures that might be necessary.
5. Plan the allocation of aspirated material to fixed slides, dried slides, cell blocks, and other studies.
6. Cleanse the skin with alcohol (briefly, as for venipuncture).
7. Perform the aspiration, with special attention to the tactile characteristics of the lesion when it is entered by the needle.
8. Apply pressure to the site after the aspiration.
9. Prepare the aspirated material.
10. Note the gross characteristics of the aspirated material.
11. Always inspect the puncture site before leaving the bedside.

at each puncture. Thus, in one typical 10- to 15-minute appointment, the patient encounters the needle for only 5 to 40 seconds.

## Steps in the Aspiration Process

### Learning about the Patient's Problem

The aspiration process begins by becoming familiar with the patient's problem. This information is often supplied by the referring physician. Its accuracy and completeness may vary from referral to referral. For example, the breast or prostate masses sent for aspiration by a surgeon or urologist are often much more highly selected than those from other physicians. This may place the physician performing the aspiration in the position of being the most experienced individual to examine the patient. While this is a new role for most pathologists, we have indicated why we feel that after experience is obtained, it is a very appropriate role.

Another important factor is that masses change over time. This is certainly the case with cysts of many types. Rapid enlargement can contribute to the clinical suspicion that a mass is malignant. When a delay of several days or a few weeks separates the initial examination of benign lymphadenopathy from the aspiration appointment, the problem may resolve. Some of these patients will have received antibiotic therapy during the interval. We have had the experience of being unable to detect the indicated adenopathy by even the most careful examination. We do not aspirate these patients because aspiration is always directed at a target lesion. We do make it clear to the patient and to the referring physician that we will be glad to reevaluate the patient if adenopathy recurs.

We then review patient radiographs and laboratory studies where appropriate. In the case of breast cytology, the mammograms can be helpful. As made clear in the literature, a benign or inconclusive cytologic result does not obviate the need for further study of a patient with mammographic or clinical abnormalities indicative of possible malignancy.[14-16] While not necessarily expert in diagnostic radiology, the physician performing the aspiration must always be aware of the radiographic findings and may frequently need to consult the radiologist. Other instances in which radiologic findings are very important include soft tissue and bone masses, as well as abdominal and hepatic tumors.

The next step in the FNA process is examination of the target lesion. When first meeting the patient, a moment should be taken to offer a greeting by name. A look at his or her face will tell much about the emotional state with which the upcoming procedure is anticipated.

A great deal of valuable information can be gained by careful physical examination. The palpatory findings in the breast may be very different for diffuse fibrocystic change, fibroadenoma, and most carcinomas. The very firm, bosselated parotid mixed tumors do not feel the same as soft, smooth, often cystic Warthin's tumors. The softness of a benign hyperplastic lymph node is different from the very hard consistency of many nodes with Hodgkin's disease, tuberculosis, or metastatic carcinoma; and the rubbery nodes of some malignant lymphomas present yet another sensation. Thus, the findings at physical examination add another set of criteria to ensure accurate and complete diagnosis. In particular, such findings can occasionally alert the microscopist that a seemingly benign specimen is inadequate, in that it is not representative of the process strongly suggested by clinical findings.

Care must be taken to ensure that the area aspirated corresponds to that chosen by the referring physician, or that the reason another area was selected is clearly documented. This is rarely a problem except in the case of extensive fibrocystic change of the breast. Later in this chapter we will illustrate some useful ways of describing puncture location.

Regardless of the quality or quantity of information supplied by the referring physician, we find it very useful to know what the patient thinks about the mass, and we usually elicit his or her description. For example, the patient who points with one finger to a breast mass is much more likely to have a significant lesion than the one who uses the palm of the hand or all of the fingertips together (usually in a circular motion) to indicate a large area of abnormality (or even the entire breast).

On the other hand, patient descriptions may be incorrect. We have usually encountered this in the setting of a long-ignored, obviously malignant breast mass. Patients will say that they only noticed it a few days ago or that it is getting smaller. In such instances, the unequivocal diagnosis of malignancy provided by FNA will often be the most rapid means by which the referring physician can break the wall of psychological denial and thus help the patient to begin dealing with the problem of malignancy.

### Planning the Aspiration

Next begins the process of planning the aspiration. Using strategies to be described subsequently, the lesion must be stabilized and held immobile. At the same time, some consideration must be given to the comfort of both the patient and the aspirator.

Selection of needle size is discussed in Chapter 1. We usually begin with a 25- (0.5 mm) or 27-gauge (0.4 mm) needle, while others prefer the 23 gauge (0.6 mm). Progression to a larger size may be helpful in rare, extensively fibrous masses, such as soft-tissue fibromatoses.

The number of punctures to be performed varies with the clinical situation. The cone-shaped biopsy volumes accessible to one needle pass (see Figure 1.14) can be expanded by multiple passes, as shown in Figure 2.1. In this way, even large areas of fibrocystic change in the breast can be sampled thoroughly. An effort is made to pass the needle through all areas of the palpable abnormality. Large malignant tumors are often aspirated two or more times, to evaluate the spectrum of microscopic findings that may be seen in such cases. On the other hand, metastatic deposits in patients with known malignancy or primary tumors of small size can often be adequately assessed with one puncture. Implicit in this statement is the knowledge that multiple smears can often be prepared from one aspiration (see Chapter 1). Also, the gross inspection of aspirated material should impart the impression of malignancy if the procedure is to be terminated after one puncture. We find this approach very useful in patients with disseminated malignancy, for whom their disease or the procedure is a source of pain.

When more than one puncture is planned, we try to inform the patient of this before the first aspiration. For the patient to have expected additional punctures cancelled when the first yields adequate material is a pleasant and welcome surprise. Being asked to allow second or third punctures when only one was expected is always unwelcome.

Another factor that affects the number of punctures needed is the time elapsed during each aspiration. Some operators leave the needle in place only briefly, while others persist for up to 10 to 20 seconds. In most aspirations, the greatest pain derives from puncture of the skin. Deeper tissues are often much less sensitive. For this reason, we often persist in aspirating for several seconds at each

Figure 2.1.
*This diagram illustrates the way in which multiple, overlapping cone-shaped aspiration volumes can encompass the entirety of a large mass. This is especially applicable to areas of fibrocystic change in the breast.*

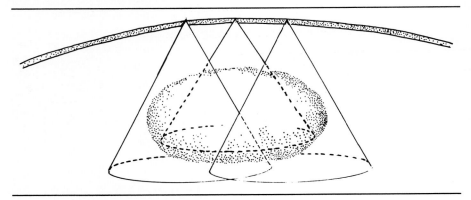

puncture and thereby are able to perform a smaller total number of aspirations. The length of the aspiration is to some extent governed by the nature and quantity of material recovered, as discussed in Chapter 1.

It is occasionally difficult to decide how many punctures will suffice to exclude a diagnosis of malignancy within the accepted limits of the FNA method. Some neoplasms are too small to be sampled confidently; others may be obscured by abnormal but benign tissue masses or cysts; still others may be very fibrous and may give up few diagnostic cells. These and other considerations give FNA a small, irreducible false-negative rate.

When special studies are likely to be necessary, planned allocation of the specimen to the various fixatives and media required can occur at this time. In a majority of cases, only good-quality smears will be needed. We do not hesitate to repeat the aspiration if the need for special studies becomes apparent after initial smear examination. The ability to do so is one of the benefits of FNA. The most common setting in which this occurs is the need for microbiologic culture of masses shown cytologically to be purulent or granulomatous.

## Implementing the Aspiration

The actual aspiration procedure usually begins by cleansing the skin with alcohol. Some prefer to use iodine-containing solutions and an elaborate preparation such as that commonly employed for bone-marrow aspiration or lumbar puncture. We prefer alcohol, used in the manner of the phlebotomist. With this technique, aspiration-site infections are virtually unheard-of. A case could be made for more elaborate skin preparation for aspiration of immunosuppressed patients or for joint aspirations. The latter is common for rheumatologists but not common for the cytopathologist.

We rarely use local anesthesia for FNA with 25- or 23-gauge needles. Local anesthesia is discussed more fully at the end of this section.

Many patients seem surprised and a bit upset when they see the pistol-like syringe holder. The size of this instrument is in marked contrast to the delicacy of FNA, as it will have been explained. For this reason, we try to keep this instrument out of the patient's field of vision. When this is not possible, we tell the patient that this instrument is for our convenience and underscore the fact that nothing will touch him or her except the examiner's fingertips and the very thin needle. When moving the syringe pistol from a nearby table to the bedside, the patient will usually not observe it at all if the physician takes that moment to look at and speak to him or her.

Issues of patient positioning are discussed later in this chapter, as aspiration of particular body sites is considered. The puncture is then executed, according to the method discussed in detail in Chapter 1. The use of multiple needle passes for larger lesions was illustrated in Figure 2.1. The range of motion (and the size of each cone of sampled tissue) varies with different anatomic sites. An aspiration volume used for large areas of thickening in the breast would clearly be inappropriate in the thyroid, for example. With very small nodules, the needle will go in and out but will move laterally only very slightly, so that the cone is extremely narrow.

As noted in Chapter 1, a split focus of vision should be developed for use during the FNA procedure. This allows simultaneous visual monitoring of the needle hub for return of material and of the patient's face for signs of distress. When the latter signs are noted, reassurance and a description of the procedure in progress may help the patient relax. This will both minimize discomfort and improve cooperation with the physician. Better-quality material, a more rapid procedure, and a less traumatized patient will result.

Just as physical examination provides clues to the possible nature of the lesion to be studied, the consistency of the mass as it is entered with the needle is also an important source of information. Most breast carcinomas are much more firm and gritty than areas of fibrocystic change, which tend to be rubbery or doughy. Many malignant lymph nodes are much more firm than their benign counterparts. When masses are deeply located (for example, in a large breast or in the abdomen), the feeling of increased resistance as the lesion is punctured can be very helpful in being sure that the mass has been entered and the situation depicted in Figure 1.2 is avoided.

At the conclusion of the aspiration, we press a gauze pad over the puncture site. In most instances, we can ask the patient to hold it in place with gentle pressure. It is very uncommon to have any bleeding after the time required to make smears of the aspirated material (usually less than 1 minute) has elapsed. If bleeding does persist, a few minutes of pressure are always sufficient to achieve hemostasis. Additional aspirations are then performed, as needed. By these simple means, FNA can be safely performed even in patients with coagulopathies.

The aspirator is occasionally surprised to see a swelling, discolored area develop immediately after breast FNA. This problem can be related to numerous large veins that are present throughout this organ. Surgeons describe occasional incidents of considerable blood loss after severing such a vein. Pressure will suffice to limit the bleeding at the time of FNA. A small bruise will result.

### Before Leaving the Patient

The final step in Table 2.3 is one to which we attach considerable importance. Before leaving the bedside, we always recheck the puncture site for bleeding or swelling and always inquire as to the patient's comfort. Problems are extremely rare, but this small amount of additional time given to the patient is often much appreciated. Care must be taken with the elderly, the weak, and those given to fainting. They must never be left unattended in a situation where a syncope- or weakness-related fall or other injury may occur.

## Local Anesthesia for Transcutaneous Aspiration

With rare exceptions, we do not use local anesthesia for FNA with 23- or 25-gauge needles. Most patients in a position to make such judgments agree that injection of anesthetic agents into the dermis is more painful than the aspiration itself. Some very anxious individuals, however, seem to derive some benefit from local anesthesia of the skin. Certainly the patient who requests local anesthesia should not be denied what he or she perceives to be an essential kindness.

Most find that tissues deep to the dermis are not overly tender and that FNA is much like getting an immunization injection. This indicates that they may receive more total pain from the lidocaine injection than from diagnostic puncture. Aspiration of muscles is often painful. This usually occurs when thyroid or lymph node aspiration is approached incorrectly, as noted subsequently herein. The periosteum overlying bones is also quite tender. Pain from this source most often occurs during breast aspiration from a very thin patient. Local anesthesia will not spare the patient these painful consequences of inept aspiration techniques.

Those using local anesthesia can apply it with a 30-gauge or 27-gauge needle. Anesthesia of the skin can be readily achieved, but it is not possible to deaden completely such masses as large areas of fibrocystic change within the breast. (As noted previously, it is also usually not necessary.)

Four potential problems attend the use of local anesthesia. The most serious is an allergic reaction to these agents. Rare individuals will experience anaphylactic reactions and may proceed rapidly to cardiovascular collapse and death. The physician should always inquire about prior administration of local anesthetics. Most adults and many children will have received these drugs previously for dental work and will know themselves to be free of allergic reactions. Those not possessing the experience and equipment to deal with severe reactions should probably not administer local anesthetic agents to individuals who have not previously received them and been free of any reaction.

The second problem is much less serious but can be distressing for the patient who expects anesthesia to remove the pain of cutaneous puncture. One occasionally discovers vials of these agents that simply seem not to work and thus provide no anesthesia. Replacing this material with a new vial from a different manufacturer's lot number will usually solve this problem.

The third problem relates to the volume of liquid injected. If too much is used in a single location, it may form a soft tissue area of firmness that is distinctly palpable and obscures the small lesion for which the patient needs FNA. This problem afflicts the neophyte who uses too much medication in an attempt to achieve a degree of anesthesia that is both impossible and unnecessary.

The last difficulty also occurs with overzealous injection of too large a volume of local anesthetic liquid. These fluids can cause morphologic distortion of cells in the mass under study and dilution of the specimen in a relatively large amount of clear liquid. We reiterate that this usually occurs when the physician attempts to create a degree of anesthesia that is both impossible and unnecessary.

Finally, we would like to offer some observations on two types of masses that are often tender, even before FNA. Granulomatous thyroiditis and some cases of fibrocystic breast thickening are often quite tender. This symptom typifies the benign character of these lesions. The patient will describe the pain, and palpation by the physician also causes pain. It is paradoxical that this pain is not increased by the needle puncture. Penetration of the skin causes brief sharp pain, but movement of the needle within the mass is not as unpleasant as palpation by the fingertips.

## ASPIRATION OF PARTICULAR BODY SITES

### General Considerations in Patient Positioning

Most aspirations are best performed with the patient supine. Not only is this the most comfortable and relaxing position, but it also eliminates the danger of an accidental fall. Another advantage is that it limits movement, should the patient be overly startled by the needle puncture. We have on one occasion seen an attack of angina pectoris immediately after prostatic aspiration. On another occasion, a patient exhibited seizure-like activity, with brief loss of consciousness, following parotid aspiration. One would prefer that such events not occur when the patient is sitting up or standing. On the other hand, if congestive heart failure is a problem, one should not put the patient in a fully recumbent position.

The general goal of positioning is to provide good access to the target lesion, with maximum comfort for the patient. (Special situations, with special goals and positioning requirements, are described subsequently.) It is an unavoidable fact of clinical medicine that some lesions simply cannot be adequately located in a supine patient. Thus, if the procedure must be performed with the patient sitting on the bed or examining table, we usually station an assistant behind the patient to provide support, should fainting occur. This is very rare, but a serious fall would be a very unfortunate complication of a supposedly benign procedure.

## Techniques for Thyroid Aspiration

### General Approach to Thyroid Aspiration

The basic anatomic relationships of the thyroid are summarized in Figure 2.2. Most of this organ's bulk lies along the posterolateral angle of the trachea, in a gutter formed by the trachea medially and by the sternocleidomastoid muscle laterally. Thus, while little tissue intervenes between the examining fingertips at

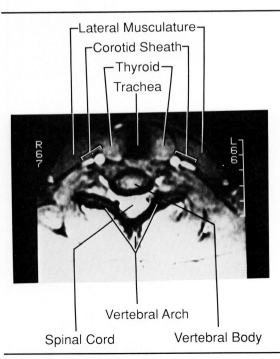

Figure 2.2.
*Nuclear magnetic resonance scan of the neck, showing the basic anatomic relationships of the thyroid. (Photograph courtesy of Dr. John Knoedler, Hennepin County Medical Center, Minneapolis, Minnesota)*

Lateral Musculature
Corotid Sheath
Thyroid
Trachea
Vertebral Arch
Spinal Cord
Vertebral Body

the skin surface and the gland itself, deep palpation may be needed to ensure adequate localization of all but the largest thyroid masses.

Most clinicians initially approach the thyroid by standing behind the patient and placing the fingertips of each hand in the anatomic gutters just described. This approach facilitates comparisons between the two lobes and will help locate small lesions, but it is not useful for the aspiration itself.

In many normal individuals, little or no thyroid tissue is palpable. The thyroid isthmus crosses the midline and is attached to tracheal rings 2 through 4. Thus, when the patient swallows, the thyroid rises and falls with other neck structures. In this way, the gland substance passes under the fingertips, and nodules become much more easily palpable. Many patients find repetitive swallowing with the physician's fingertips on the neck somewhat difficult. This effort will frequently be aided by encouraging the patient to take small sips of water in order to initiate swallowing.

Once the mass has been localized, we then make note of its position for our report. This can be done with a drawing of the neck or with a verbal description. We describe the side on which a mass occurs, as well as whether it is nearer the upper or the lower pole. A few masses will be in the midline at the level of the isthmus. It is difficult to accurately describe the location of thyroid nodules in reference to external landmarks such as the sternal notch. This is because distances between structures in the neck appear to change, depending on whether the cervical spine is in flexion or extension.

Figure 2.3 shows the preferred position for most thyroid aspirations. When a pillow is placed under the shoulders, the cervical spine is put into extension. This places the soft tissue overlying the thyroid in a stretched position and thins them as much as possible. Of course, if too much tension is placed on the skin of the neck, it will be stretched too tight to allow detailed palpation of the thyroid. A balance must be achieved by adjusting the pillow under the patient's shoulders. This position also thrusts the larynx and upper trachea anteriorly and superiorly, bringing with them the thyroid. We find that this positioning maximizes the ease with which small thyroid nodules can be located and aspirated.

Recalling the anatomy in Figure 2.2, it is apparent that the needle should be angled slightly toward the midline. In this way, it is actually being directed toward the trachea and the vertebral bones, and away from the carotid sheath and its vascular contents. Furthermore, with the palpating fingertips between the trachea and the sternocleidomastoid muscle, the muscle is pushed laterally and out of the needle's path. Thyroid aspirations that contain abundant skeletal muscle have usually been obtained improperly. Vigorous sampling of skeletal muscle is often painful and should be avoided.

When the needle is directed medially, the only structure likely to be inadvertently punctured is the trachea. When this happens, air will enter the syringe so that suction is lost and the aspiration must be initiated again. In this manner, tracheal mucosal cells and mucus may occasionally be seen on the thyroid FNA smears (Figure 2.4). In elderly patients, tracheal cartilage is often ossified and may contain fat and bone marrow. When marrow elements are aspirated unexpectedly, the immature granulocytes and large hyperchromatic megakaryocytes may be confused with cells of a malignancy (Figure 2.5). Despite the surprise experienced at tracheal puncture when syringe vacuum is suddenly

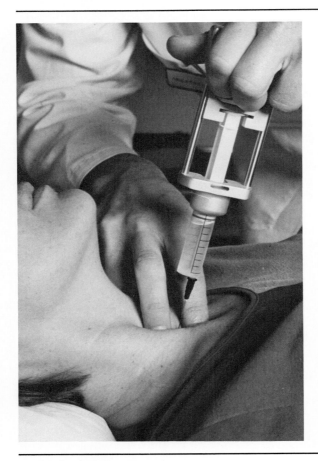

Figure 2.3.
*The preferred position for most thyroid aspirations is shown here. A pillow is placed under the patient's shoulders. This puts the cervical spine in extension, thereby thinning the soft tissues overlying the thyroid. Note that the needle is directed medially and sternocleidomastoid muscle is displaced laterally as the two fingertips stabilize the mass. See text for additional description.*

lost or when ciliated cells, mucus, or bone marrow elements are seen on smears thought to be from the thyroid, the most important thing to note is that no adverse consequences attend the tracheal puncture.

### Cystic Thyroid Aspirations

Many thyroid nodules are cystic or partially cystic and can be evacuated by needle aspiration. Because vigorous needle motion can cause bleeding, some of these may refill with blood almost immediately after evacuation unless the aspiration is very gentle. For this reason, we puncture the nodule with a single smooth motion and await a fluid return while holding the needle stationary within the mass. If none appears, we then progress to a very gentle, low-amplitude needle motion. Many thyroid lesions are highly vascular, and this type of motion will suffice to obtain a specimen with minimal blood.

When cyst fluid is obtained, it should be processed by centrifugation. We usually keep it in the syringe and use a clean needle with its plastic cap in place to seal the fluid in the syringe. After cyst evacuation, a careful repeat examination should be directed at the detection of any residual mass. If present, this mass should be the target of repeat aspiration.

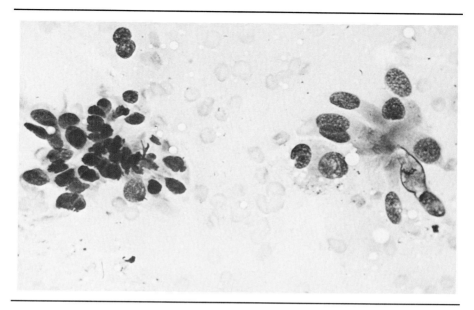

Figure 2.4.
*The ciliated columnar cells and the mucus of tracheal origin were obtained when the trachea was punctured during thyroid aspiration (modified Diff-Quik® stain, ×160 before a 28% reduction).*

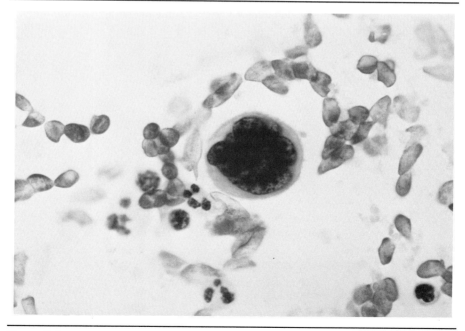

Figure 2.5.
*Bone-marrow cells, including large megakaryocytes, may be seen in smears from ossified tracheal cartilage that have been punctured during thyroid aspiration (Papanicolaou stain, ×788 before a 34% reduction).*

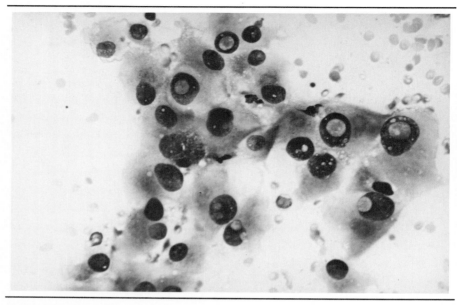

Figure 2.6.
*Concentrated fluid from a cystic papillary carcinoma of the thyroid. The tumor cells are large, with dense cytoplasm, sharp cell borders, large nuclei, and frequent intranuclear cytoplasmic inclusions (modified Diff Quik® stain, ×312 before a 28% reduction).*

Most thyroid cyst fluids represent benign lesions, but some degree of cystic degeneration is common in papillary carcinoma. One study found an incidence of cystic change of almost 17 percent.[17] Figure 2.6 shows an example of cystic papillary carcinoma. The background cyst fluid contains red cells and foamy macrophages. The tumor-cell groups, though few in number, are quite distinctive and show typical features of papillary carcinoma. Cystic change can also occur in follicular carcinomas.[18]

Although up to 20 percent of nonfunctioning thyroid nodules are cysts and the majority of such lesions are benign, a fluid containing only red cells and macrophages can never be designated as unequivocally benign because the lining epithelium responsible for the cyst has not been sampled. Any residual mass should be aspirated, as should any cyst recurrence. Approaches to the diagnosis of such cases range from calling them "unsatisfactory" to describing them as "nondiagnostic."[17] Whichever term is used, they should not be called "negative." Such a benign diagnosis ignores the fact that occasional nondiagnostic cyst fluids will have originated in a carcinoma. On the other hand, patients with a long history of thyroid enlargement, a family history of goiter, bilateral disease or multinodular enlargement have a low probability of malignancy and may be conservatively managed. The malignancy most likely to be present in a cyst fluid is papillary carcinoma. No harm will result from a delay in diagnosis resulting from conservative management of a nondiagnostic thyroid-cyst evacuation.

*Clinical Goals of Thyroid Aspiration*

For many physicians in North America, it is in the thyroid that the goals and utility of FNA are most clearly defined. Nonfunctioning nodular goiter is very common, affecting 4 to 7 percent of the population.[19] Thyroid malignancy, on the other hand, is very uncommon and constitutes 0.5 percent of all malignancies and 5 percent of patients referred for evaluation of a thyroid nodule.[20] FNA can accurately distinguish neoplastic from nonneoplastic lesions in most cases. The very large number of patients with nonneoplastic lesions do not usually require surgery. (Nodular goiter is occasionally treated surgically when the bulk of thyroid tissue is sufficiently great to cause difficulties due to compression of the trachea or other vital structures.)

Silverman et al. described aspirations from 309 patients, of whom only 60 were treated surgically. Of these 60 patients, 72 percent of the resected lesions were neoplastic. This very high surgical yield was possible because most nonneoplastic lesions were excluded from surgery by preoperative cytologic diagnosis.[21] The most cost-effective and efficient algorithms for evaluation of thyroid masses begin with needle aspiration.[22] This approach is so successful that some large institutions have virtually stopped using thyroid radioisotope scans and ultrasonography for the initial workup of thyroid masses. These expensive techniques often contribute little to the distinction of benign from malignant mass lesions.[23,24]

In other studies, introduction of FNA reduced thyroid surgery from 63 to 43 percent of patients and increased the operative finding of carcinoma from 14 to 29 percent.[23,25] In a series studied by Hawkins et al., the percentage of patients undergoing surgery decreased from 61 to 14 percent, while the recovery of malignancies increased from 8.3 to 37.3 percent.[26] Thus, while cytopathologists pursue the study of thyroid neoplasms, the usual goal of thyroid FNA is identification of the few cases that require surgery. Most thyroid enlargements do not require surgery for either diagnosis or therapy.

# Techniques for Breast Aspiration

Those physicians seeing the broad spectrum of patients who require FNA will spend up to 80 percent of their aspiration clinic time engaged in the study of breast lesions. This extremely important area is given great attention in the literature on FNA interpretation. Just as important, however, is the proper clinical approach to the patient. Because of its importance and the ubiquity of its study, we have used the breast as an example of techniques and problems throughout our discussion.

*Diagnostic Approaches to Breast Lesions*

Surgical procedures excluded, there are four techniques commonly used to evaluate breast masses: physical examination, FNA cytology, mammography, and ultrasonography. In the case of palpable masses, the contemporary approach features FNA as soon as a lesion is detected. Other studies are then less urgent but are needed for evaluation of normal-appearing areas in the ipsilateral breast, as well as the contralateral one. (Aspiration of nonpalpable, mammographically detected lesions is a highly specialized subject beyond the scope of this book.)

In each case, the purpose is to diagnose malignancies preoperatively and to identify and safely follow patients with benign disease. Because up to 50 percent of women have some element of fibrocystic change, it is not possible to biopsy surgically all diffusely lumpy breasts.[27] Therefore, we direct each of these diagnostic modalities as skillfully as possible, to detect breast malignancy and to identify women likely to harbor high-risk marker lesions.[28]

The accuracy of each diagnostic modality varies from series to series. From 8 to 38 percent of breast carcinomas are not detected by palpation alone. When mammography is added to the physical examination, up to 85 percent are detected preoperatively. By adding FNA, 93 to 100 percent are identified.[9,14,29] In Kreuzer and Boquoi's series, concordance of the three methods indicated results that were correct more than 99 percent of the time. It is important that each step be carried out by an expert in the area. As we have previously noted, we feel that many mistakes in FNA happen at the bedside rather than at the microscope.

Physical examination of the breast requires a great deal of experience to perfect. Furthermore, results are plagued by some degree of subjectivism; not all observers will agree about subtle findings. It is very important that the patient's perception of masses, thickenings, or discomfort be elicited and taken seriously. Techniques for describing and recording the precise location of breast lesions are discussed subsequently in the section on evaluation of breast carcinoma.

### Approach to Evaluation of Breast Cytology

Most writers about breast cytology indicate the microscopic pitfalls. False-negative diagnoses can occur due to poor technique, inaccurate interpretation, or failure to recognize a well-differentiated type of malignancy. Some breast carcinomas are extremely sclerotic, and their dense fibrous stroma precludes aspiration of highly cellular material. As mentioned previously, this hypocellularity is a diagnostic clue to infiltrating carcinoma of the lobular type and to purely intraductal carcinoma. Some false negatives are inevitable when densely fibrous malignancies are studied.

Referring to the ground rules mentioned in Table 2.2, it is clear that in the face of clinical or mammographic evidence of possible malignancy, the problem is left unsolved by such an aspiration, and another diagnostic test (usually surgical excision) must be performed. This illustrates the importance of combining all clinical, radiographic, and cytologic findings in total patient care. This is one of the reasons given in Table 2.1 for preferring to concentrate the aspiration procedure in the hands of a single individual who does many procedures and who will evaluate the cytologic material in the light of clinical findings. Our comments in the previous section on "who should perform aspirations" have particular relevance to the study of breast lesions.

The cytopathologist should not rely too heavily on the mammogram. The primary utility of this test is identification of nonpalpable lesions. When a palpable mass is present, FNA should be the first-line diagnostic method. Mammography is then used to study nonpalpable disease in both breasts.

Approximately 10 to 15 percent of palpable breast carcinomas will not be visualized by mammography. This in no way decreases the value or accuracy of a cytologic diagnosis of malignancy.

Cytologic pitfalls that may lead to false-positive diagnoses have been described. Some—such as pregnancy, lactation, or traumatic fat necrosis—can be avoided if accurate historical information is coupled with careful consideration of microscopic findings. The atypical fibroadenoma can be suspected if the patient has been examined by the microscopist. Still others, such as certain reparative stromal reactions and the granular cell tumor, can only be successfully diagnosed if considerable expertise is brought to the microscopy.

Histopathologists recognize a host of firm, stellate breast lesions that are benign but can clinically, radiographically, and histologically mimic carcinoma. These are summarized in Table 2.4.[30-36] Keen, et al. reviewed their experience with benign breast masses that clinically and mammographically appeared malignant. Their nine cases included examples of indurative mastopathy, sclerosing papillary proliferation, infarcted papilloma, sclerosing adenosis, and fat necrosis.[30]

A recitation of such conditions that may be mistaken for carcinoma often goes through the mind of the surgical pathologist who is called upon to diagnose breast carcinoma intraoperatively with frozen section material. A similar mental approach must be taken with FNA specimens. Carcinoma must be diagnosed with certainty only when multiple cytologic criteria are met. While suspicion of malignancy on clinical or mammographic grounds is sufficient to lead to a biopsy, neither is sufficient to result in an FNA diagnosis of carcinoma when it is not cytologically inescapable. Neither the radiologists' feeling that a given lesion may represent cancer nor the surgeon's being "sure that it is cancer" constitutes a reason to diagnose carcinoma when the cytologic findings are not compelling.

## Special Problems in Breast Aspiration

Several of these are summarized in Table 2.5.

*Cysts*    A special problem is the handling of fluids aspirated from breast cysts. Less than 3 percent of cysts are associated with a malignancy.[14,37,38] Their sig-

Table 2.4

*Firm, stellate benign breast lesions that may simulate carcinoma clinically, mammographically, and histologically*

Sclerosing papillary proliferation
Nonencapsulated sclerosing lesion
Indurative mastopathy
Radial scar
Fibromatosis
Fat necrosis
Elastosis in benign ductal proliferations
Granular cell tumor
Infarcted papilloma
Florid sclerosing adenosis

Table 2.5
*Problems requiring a careful approach to aspiration of palpable breast lesions*

1. Large, ill-defined areas of thickening require multiple overlapping aspirations. Even so, some sampling error is inevitable. Small malignancies may be obscured by fibrosis and cysts.

2. Small mobile breast masses require great skill for accurate puncture.

3. Many breast masses are deeper than they feel. Care must be taken to use a needle of sufficient length and to attend to the feeling of the needle entering the lesion.

4. Some patients are referred with multiple areas of increased density. Each must be considered as a separate aspiration event, and each may require more than one puncture.

5. In patients with small breasts, the needle may at times be quite close to the pleural surface. Pneumothorax is rare but has been described.

6. Aspirations involving the skin of the nipple and areola can be very painful for the patient.

nificance is that they may conceal a malignancy from physical or radiographic examinations. Many surgeons aspirate cysts in the office and are accustomed to discarding the fluid rather than submitting it for cytologic examination. With the typical pale yellow or light green fluid in most cysts, this is an acceptable practice. If, however, the fluid is turbid or bloody, it should be centrifuged and examined microscopically. Fluids obtained from cysts that recur rapidly after drainage should also be examined microscopically.

Frable recommends the following steps in cyst evaluation: (1) Evacuate the cyst completely. (2) Carefully reexamine the patient for any residual mass in the area of the cyst. If any is found, it should be aspirated as any other breast mass. (3) Repeat the mammography to look for any suspicious areas that might have been obscured by the cyst. (4) Process the fluid, and examine it microscopically, if indicated.[2]

*Large Ill-Defined Breast Thickenings*   Many patients are referred for evaluation of breast lesions that are of very low suspicion for malignancy. Historical and physical clues to the nature of benign fibrocystic change should be sought. These lesions are often areas of prominence or asymmetry in breasts that are diffusely lumpy or thickened. Focal thickenings or asymmetry between the two breasts may be reflected in the mammogram. These radiographs will frequently confirm the abnormality but show no features suggestive of a malignant process. Such masses may be ill-defined on physical examination. Unless distinct, rounded cysts are present, the lesion may be difficult to delineate, as its borders fade into the surrounding tissue.

The patient will often indicate the area of abnormality with several fingers or with a broad circular motion of the hand. This is very different from the patient who points to a discrete mass with the tip of one finger. The latter lesion is more likely to feel like a cyst, a fibroadenoma, or a malignancy. Benign lesions are more frequently tender or painful than are malignancies. The patient may describe changes of the mass with her menstrual cycle. She may have gained some symptomatic relief by a caffeine-free diet.

Because such areas of thickening are very common, not all of these cases can be reasonably approached surgically. In some patients, however, such thickenings will obscure areas of malignancy. The addition of FNA to physical examination and mammography will increase the preoperative identification of malignancy and will increase the physician's confidence in nonsurgical follow-up of benign disease.

Adequate sampling is of paramount importance in these lesions but is difficult to define. A method of multiple, overlapping, cone-shaped aspiration volumes, as illustrated in Figure 2.1, is the best approach to larger thickenings in the breast. We generally perform a minimum of three thorough aspirations in such cases, but more may be needed in some instances. While it is difficult to say how many are enough, it is usually clear that one is insufficient. While we always try to perform thorough, careful aspirations, the fact that this technique (like any other sampling method) has a small, seemingly irreducible false-negative rate remains. With this in mind, neither the quality of the procedure nor the thoroughness of patient follow-up can be allowed to diminish.

*Small Mobile Lumps*    The second problem described in Table 2.5 is that small, mobile breast lumps make very challenging targets for FNA. These are among the most technically difficult of all aspiration procedures. The techniques for stabilizing masses with the fingers of the left hand, which were described in Chapter 1, are very useful in this situation. Figure 2.7 shows that the technique changes as the size of the mass is reduced. In the case of very small masses, the lesion can be held securely beneath the tip of the index finger. When the mass is pressed beneath the fingertip and the finger is moved back and forth over a short distance, the mobile tumor can be felt to slip past the fingertip (Figure 2.8).

It is often helpful to perform the aspiration with the nodule in the position indicated by Figure 2.9. It can be held against the fingertip. As mentioned in Chapter 1, the mass can be thought of as an extension of the nondominant hand's

Figure 2.7.
*Methods of stabilizing palpable masses vary with the size of the mass. Large or midsized lesions can be held between two fingers. Small masses can be located beneath the tip of the index finger.*

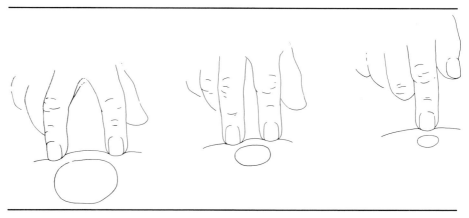

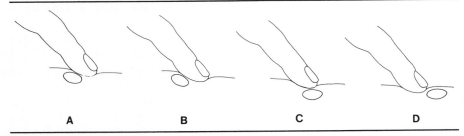

**Figure 2.8.**
*When a small nodule is pressed beneath the tip of the index finger, and the fingertip is moved over the mass (A–D), it can be felt to slip past the fingertip.*

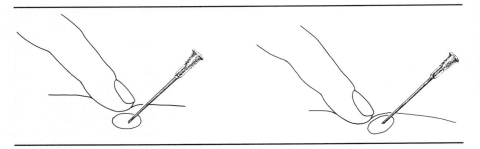

**Figure 2.9.**
*(A) The small nodule can be held beneath the tip of the index finger. (B) When the fingertip is moved back and forth, the nodule will remain stable, having been fixed in place by the needle. Thus, it will not be felt to roll beneath the moving fingertip, as in Figure 2.8.*

index finger. With the needle acting as an extension of the dominant hand, the accurate puncture of small nodules becomes conceptually like touching the tips of the physician's two index fingers together. When the nodule has been entered by the needle (Figure 2.9), the fingertip can again be moved back and forth in an attempt to repeat the maneuver shown in Figure 2.8. If held in place by the needle, the nodule will be stationary and will not be felt rolling under the fingertip. Furthermore, the very thin and flexible 25- or 27-gauge needle will bend freely as pressure is applied to the nodule. This is very helpful in being sure that small nodules have been penetrated accurately. This technique can be applied not only to breast nodules but also to a variety of small palpable lesions in many sites, such as lymph nodes.

*Deep Seated Breast Masses*    As illustrated in Figure 1.2, many breast masses are deeper than initial physical examination may suggest. Those new to performing aspirations begin to learn this when lesions that are highly suspicious for malignancy (that is, well defined and very firm) yield scant nondiagnostic smears. The way in which this problem can be overcome is by feeling the lesion carefully with the needle tip. This will usually suffice to ensure that the mass has been penetrated during the aspiration. In the patient with very large breasts, one must also be careful to use a needle of sufficient length. A 25-gauge (0.5 mm) needle of 1 1/2 inch (3.8 cm) length is usually acceptable. On rare occasions, we have used a needle of 2-inch (5 cm) length.

*Multiple Masses*    Some patients are referred for evaluation of multiple areas of increased density that may involve both breasts. Each of these must be considered separately. Each may require more than one aspiration. Each lesion should be described, localized, and reported separately. Techniques for describing and recording the precise location of breast lesions are discussed in the section on aspiration of carcinomas.

*Complications of Breast Puncture*    A discussion of bleeding due to puncture of the large veins of the breast was presented earlier in this chapter. The patient with very small breasts presents a special problem. The needle tip can come very close to the chest-wall soft tissues or even to the pleura. The danger is that a pneumothorax can occur if the pleura is punctured. This complication is rare but has been reported. One multi-institutional study described 74,000 breast aspirations performed with 21- to 23-gauge needles. Thirteen (0.018%) instances of pneumothorax were noted. None was severe, and none required chest-tube placement for treatment.[39] In this series, pneumothorax caused sudden thoracic pain without dyspnea. (As noted in the section on lymph-node aspiration, pneumothorax is also a potential complication of axillary or supraclavicular aspirations.) To avoid this difficulty, breast lesions of this type should be entered with the needle oriented tangentially rather than perpendicular to the skin surface.

*Painful Aspiration of Masses Near the Nipple*    Retroareolar masses can be a problem because the skin of the nipple and areola tends to be very sensitive to pain. Because the retroareolar soft tissues are also sensitive, some pain is often unavoidable. The kindest thing that we can do in this situation is to perform the aspiration skillfully and rapidly. To avoid the areolar skin, the retroareolar area can be entered tangentially. Another solution is to push the mass out from beneath the areolar area so that it can be aspirated through skin at some distance from this complex. Figure 2.10 shows one way to accomplish this.

### Aspiration of the Male Breast

Aspiration of the male breast is occasionally required. A tangential approach is often favored, to avoid having the needle come close to the pleura. We have encountered clear-cut carcinomas of the male breast, but these are uncommon. The most often encountered palpable lesion is gynecomastia. This may be unilateral or bilateral and is sometimes tender to palpation. The typical case presents as a round, symmetrical, disclike or platelike retroareolar thickening that is mobile. It may be central or eccentric.

The histopathology of gynecomastia explains the aspiration results. As shown in Figure 2.11, the histology is characterized by distended ducts, with or without lobular development. The ducts are separated by dense fibrous stroma that is pale and edematous in the periductal areas. The ductal epithelium shows varying degrees of hyperplasia, with multiple cell layers and papillary architecture.

When aspirated, these lesions are very dense and feel rubbery with the needle.

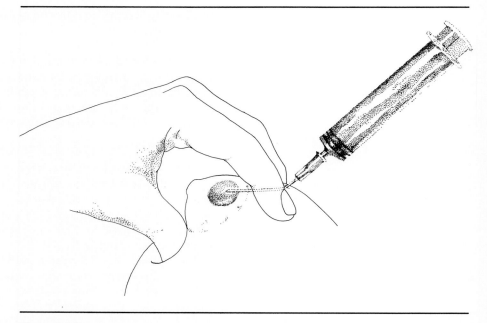

Figure 2.10.
*This retroareolar mass has been pushed by the thumb out from under the areolar skin.*
*This will allow it to be punctured through skin that is much less sensitive to pain than that*
*of the nipple–areola complex. The mass is held stable between the thumb on one side and*
*the two fingers on the other side.*

Considerable force is sometimes required to move the needle in and out through
the fibrous stroma. A small amount of fluid may be obtained, reflecting the
periductal edema. Because the ducts are widely separated, the amount of ductal
epithelium that is aspirated depends on its proliferative activity and on the
thoroughness of the procedure. Both flat sheets and papillary groups can be
obtained, and either may show considerable cytologic atypia.

The surgical pathologist's conservative approach to papillary lesions occur-
ring in the nipple and areola should extend to the interpretation of cytologic
material. Furthermore, even more conservatism is in order when the male breast
is studied. The diagnosis of malignancy should be reserved for those occasions
on which the morphologic and clinical evidence is truly overwhelming.

Gynecomastia is often a reflection of hyperestrinism. Thus, while many cases
are idiopathic, this condition can be a reflection of other disease states. Table 2.6
summarizes some of the clinical settings in which gynecomastia occurs.[40,41]
Questioning the patient along these lines will often provide historical information that supports the cytologic and physical impression of gynecomastia. Also,
this brief bit of history taking may contribute to a more complete evaluation of
the patient's problem.

Aspiration of gynecomastia is often very painful. Many men find the procedure difficult to tolerate. Skill and rapidity (without sacrifice of thoroughness)

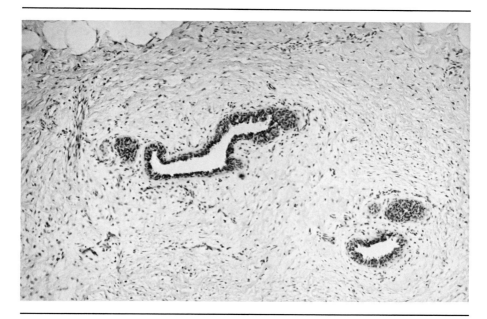

Figure 2.11.
*The histology of gynecomastia shows large ducts separated by dense fibrous tissue, periductal edema and a variable degree of ductal epithelial hyperplasia (H&E, ×125 before a 22% reduction).*

Table 2.6
*Causes of gynecomastia*

Physiologic hyperestrinism
    Puberty
    Old age (altered relation between testicular and adrenal hormone)

Pathologic hyperestrinism
    Testicular neoplasms (Leydig or Sertoli tumors)
    Cirrhosis
    Klinefelter's syndrome
    Chronic use of marijuana
    Heroin addiction
    Therapeutic drugs*
    Trauma
    Prolonged infections
    Autoimmune disorders
    Malignancies[†]
    Hyperthyroidism or hypothyroidism
    Idiopathic causes

*Digitalis, reserpine, ergotamine, testosterone, thyroid extract and diphenylhydantoin (see Reference 40).

[†]Epithelial malignancies of the prostate, colon, lung, or testis, as well as malignant lymphoma.

are important. Envisioning the area of gynecomastia as a thin, round, plate-like area of tissue behind the areola, we enter the skin tangentially some distance from the areola and then anticipate the firm feel as the needle enters the fibrous tissue. The needle is then moved back and forth and in and out in a much flattened version of the previously described cone-shaped tissue volume. Its motion is more like that of a fan-shaped distribution. This allows penetration of large areas of tissue in the medial to lateral and superior to inferior planes without close approach to the deep soft tissues and pleura.

### Aspiration of Carcinoma

Many carcinomas will be strongly suspected by clinical findings prior to FNA. Cytology can provide a firm, presurgical diagnosis of malignancy. This permits optimal counseling of the patient regarding treatment possibilities. Furthermore, preoperative diagnosis eliminates the need for two-stage surgical procedures in which separate operations are used for diagnostic biopsy and for definitive resection.

A newly evolving indication for preoperative diagnosis of breast carcinoma by FNA is neoadjuvant chemotherapy. In this type of treatment protocol, chemical treatment is administered following diagnosis by FNA. Surgery is then performed. Tumor shrinkage may improve the resectability of larger lesions. The ultimate effect on patient outcome remains to be investigated. Those evaluating patients for neoadjuvant therapy need to be cognizant of the fact that hormone receptor studies and DNA analysis must be performed on aspirated material. Special specimen handling will be necessary and should be planned either at the time of the initial study or at the time of repeat FNA, performed specifically to secure material for these studies.

When carcinomas are aspirated, they can often be felt as very firm. This perception is often described as "gritty" and is quite different from the rubbery or doughy feeling of benign breast lesions with dense fibrosis. An exception to this typical description is mucinous carcinoma, which is very soft.[42]

A similar situation occurs in medullary carcinoma because, as its name implies, this tumor is fleshy in texture and is by definition well circumscribed.[43] (When diagnosed by rigorously applied criteria, medullary carcinoma is a very uncommon entity. In FNA material, it is difficult or impossible to distinguish from poorly differentiated infiltrating carcinoma that lacks the features of medullary carcinoma.)

The aspiration of breast carcinomas frequently yields abundant material, so that several slides can be prepared from one puncture as described in Chapter 1. However, scanty smears may imply infiltrating lobular carcinoma or purely intraductal carcinoma. The hypocellular nature of the preparations mandate considerable circumspection in their microscopic interpretation.

As noted previously, many patients develop multiple breast abnormalities that may be studied by FNA. These may occur synchronously or at different times. A benign lesion in no way precludes the subsequent development of a malignancy. Thus, it is imperative that the exact site, size, and clinical characteristics of the mass under study be described for the referring physician and for ease of comparison with future studies. The traditional description of the quadrant in which the lesion is found is not sufficient for this purpose.

Two methods of location description can be used. The first is to draw and label an illustration of the clinical findings. While it is very helpful to receive such illustrations from the referring physician, they are very difficult to catalogue in the computerized archive that often characterizes record keeping in the modern laboratory. A method of permanently recording this information uses a simple system of polar coordinates, as illustrated in Figure 2.12. The data generated by this type of localization are very suitable for computerized report archives.

The exact position of a mobile lesion may change, depending on whether the patient is supine or sitting at the time of examination. As described previously, we prefer to perform most aspirations with the patient supine. Standardizing this practice further minimizes any equivocation about the precise localization of a mobile breast mass. If, however, the lesion must be aspirated with the patient sitting, this should certainly be noted in the description of its localization.

## Clinical Correlations in Breast Cytology

When clinical, radiographic, and cytologic findings are tabulated, most patients referred for cytologic evaluation of palpable abnormalities in the breast fall into one of the three categories, summarized in Table 2.7. (Patients with lesions clinically typical of cyst or fibroadenoma are not included in this tabulation.)

The first and largest group consists of patients who have breast-parenchyma thickenings that are often ill-defined and not clinically suggestive of malignancy.

Figure 2.12.
*A system of polar coordinates can be used for accurately localizing breast masses. The left breast lesion depicted here measures 2 × 3 cm, is located between 1 o'clock and 2 o'clock, and is centered 6 cm from the nipple.*

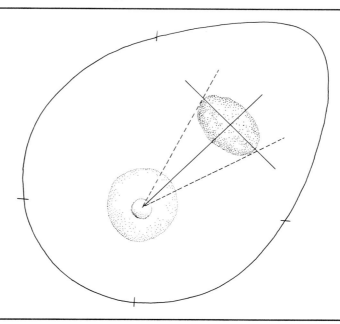

Table 2.7
*Three categories that comprise most breast FNA patients\**

|  | Clinical Findings | Mammographic Findings | FNA Findings | Incidence | Action |
|---|---|---|---|---|---|
| 1. Thickening not suspicious for malignancy | Benign | Benign | Very common | Clinical and x-ray follow-up[†] |
| 2. Mass lesion | Variable; may be negative | Cancer | Variable; may be common | Surgery |
| 3. Any one of the three modalities is atypical or is suspicious for malignancy | | | Least common | Surgery |

\*Including only patients with lesions not typical of either cyst or fibroadenoma.

[†]Unless more definitive intervention is indicated by clinical considerations or the patient's wishes.

Because not all patients with these abnormalities can undergo surgery and because fibrocystic change can conceal a malignancy, further evaluation is frequently in order. When the mammogram and the FNA are also clearly benign, the clinician gains confidence in following these lesions without immediate surgical biopsy.

As noted previously, when all these diagnostic modalities are carefully applied and each is performed and interpreted by highly qualified individuals, very few malignancies will go undiagnosed. However, there remains a small false-negative rate in the best of programs. Therefore, follow-up is also an essential part of breast evaluation. This was clearly indicated in the patient-education materials described earlier in this chapter.

The second group of patients consists of those with clear evidence of malignancy. Often, the physical examination and the cytology are both typical of carcinoma. In our experience, the aspiration is frequently performed as soon as the mass is discovered and before there is time for mammography. When the clinical and cytologic findings are clearly those of a malignant process, we do not hesitate to make that diagnosis even in the absence of radiographic studies. It is very important to continue efforts to schedule mammography, so that the contralateral breast is adequately evaluated.

The unequivocal cytologic diagnosis of carcinoma should be rendered only when multiple criteria of malignancy are satisfied. Because this includes high cellularity, the usual cases have abundant material on several slides from each of two or more punctures. We have described a case where both malignant-appearing and benign-appearing areas could be found not only on different slides but also within a single slide.[44] Thus, when features of a benign process are present, they should preclude an unequivocal diagnosis of carcinoma. The aforementioned case was excised and showed a fibroadenoma with atypia.

The final clinical subset is numerically the smallest. These are patients who have some atypia or suspicion of malignancy by one or more of the three diagnostic methods. These patients should undergo surgical biopsy. As summarized in Table 2.2, a benign cytologic report in a patient with clinical or radiographic suspicion of malignancy is in no way reassuring. Bell et al. reviewed the literature on the cytologically suspicious breast aspiration.[14] These were cases in which the cellular abnormalities fell short of the criteria for malignancy. Such smears were obtained in from 1.6 to 8.4 percent of studies. Follow-up showed that from 41 to 87 percent represented malignancy. Atypia suspicious for malignancy occurs in a few benign processes and can be due to degenerative changes, fibroadenoma,[44] papillary processes, benign proliferative lesions, and atypical hyperplasias. As discussed earlier, some proliferations that are not overtly malignant must be evaluated histologically to identify patients who are at an increased risk for subsequent development of malignancy.[27,28] The cyto-logic findings in atypical breast lesions have not yet been fully defined. At this time, all such cases should be biopsied surgically.

The suggested relative proportions of these three patient groups are typical of clinical practices that comprise a large number of breast patients; we have described the general practice of FNA. This type of practice experience generally assumes large numbers of patients referred by numerous physicians of different specialties.

Referral of patients for FNA of breast lesions is not a standardized process in North America. It varies among different localities, depending on the types of physicians in practice, the availability of FNA at regional training centers, and the quality of cytology services offered by local pathologists. Some physicians refer virtually all patients to the FNA clinic. In some instances, these individuals are seeking consultation for physical examination by a more experienced colleague. Some of their patients will not be suitable candidates for FNA. Others refer only patients who seem certain to have a breast malignancy. These physicians wish to improve preoperative counseling. Still others will refer only patients with apparently benign disease, wishing to improve the security of nonsurgical follow-up for these patients. Clearly, the cytopathologist's case mix depends heavily on referral patterns.

## Medicolegal Considerations in Breast Aspiration

The largest group of patients seen by the cytopathologist may be the first group noted in Table 2.7: These cases are referred for evaluation of breast abnormalities that do not form discrete masses or tumors of the type clinically suggestive of malignancy, cyst, or fibroadenoma. Instead, they present with areas of firmness or thickening. These areas are ill-defined and often merge gradually into the surrounding breast tissue, which itself may be diffusely lumpy. When coupled with a benign mammogram and a benign FNA report, the probability that carcinoma is present is quite low. Most clinicians will follow these patients rather than perform surgery. Follow-up will include repeated physical examination, x-ray, and FNA at appropriate intervals.

It is inevitable that rare small carcinomas will be missed by even the most careful and skillful application of this diagnostic triad. They will have been hidden from the fingertips, the x-ray film, and aspirating needle by the larger area of the fibrocystic change in which they are embedded. A small, irreducible, false-negative rate thus persists.

In the light of the foregoing discussion, it seems that the pathologist who sees the patient, takes a sample, and then makes a microscopic diagnosis has assumed a new level of medicolegal liability not previously experienced by this specialty. No body of malpractice claims has accumulated, but the potential for failure-to-diagnose-cancer or delay-in-diagnosis-of-cancer types of lawsuits is clear. The risk is probably least in malignant masses of the breast or lymph nodes from which one often recovers abundant material. It is probably greatest in these seemingly low-risk breast thickenings. In the former, one makes a diagnosis of carcinoma by identifying malignant cells. In the latter, one draws a positive conclusion ("the lesion is benign") from negative information ("no cancer cells are seen").

In most legal actions, the physician's work is cast in the best possible light only if it is clearly documented in the medical record that all appropriate actions were taken. Furthermore, the patient must have been fully informed about alternative methods of diagnosis and the potential false-negative rate. We use the type of brochure described previously to accomplish these goals. The manner in which the procedure details can be documented is discussed subsequently, in the section on results reporting. For now, suffice it to say that the report should reflect the interpreter's awareness of the clinical findings, localization of the area aspirated, thoroughness of sampling, microscopic findings, interpretation, and any suggestions for the patient's further evaluation or follow-up.

Finally, complete patient care requires adequate follow-up of those individuals with apparently benign breast lesions. When we see patients referred by experienced surgeons, this quality of follow-up is almost certain because it is a daily part of the surgeon's practice. If the referring physician is a general practitioner, gynecologist, or internist, however, some comments on appropriate follow-up may be helpful.

Thus, the cytopathologist assumes some of the role involved in a new medical specialty. Concentrating skills in physical examination and cytologic diagnosis in the hands of the FNA specialist has many benefits for the patient. Benefits also accrue to the referring physician who is less experienced in the examination and management of specialized problems such as breast masses. The practitioner should be aware that he or she may be assuming a new level of medicolegal responsibility. Adequate training, experience, and skill are required to fill this role. Careful documentation provides the best protection from the inevitable shortcomings of this (or any other) medical procedure.

## Techniques for Lymph-Node Aspiration

Lymph nodes suitable for aspiration without radiographic guidance generally present as small subcutaneous targets. Their sizes range from very small to several centimeters. The technique for obtaining material from lymph nodes is usually not different from that previously described. In the case of very small nodes, the stabilization techniques illustrated in Figures 2.7 through 2.9 are helpful.

### Aspiration Technique

Lymph nodes of the neck are commonly studied by aspiration. Many of these are small and mobile. The ease with which they can be palpated may depend on the way in which the patient is examined. Small nodes may seem to disappear into the musculature of the neck as the head is rotated or the neck is placed in either flexion or extension. One may need to ask the patient to move the head in various ways to gain free access to small nodes. Final adjustments can be made when the physician moves the patient's head slightly with the dominant hand while palpating and stabilizing the target node with the fingers of the nondominant hand.

Submandibular nodes may require bimanual palpation, with the nondominant hand inside the mouth and the dominant hand outside it. (It is much more comfortable for the patient if the gloved hand is moistened by running water before it is placed in the patient's mouth.) Inside the patient's mouth, the gloved fingers of the nondominant hand push the node inferiorly by pressing in the sulcus between the floor of the mouth and the lower, inner border of the mandible. The lymph node can then be palpated outside the patient's mouth subcutaneously, with the fingers of the dominant hand, in the usual fashion. One can then hold the node with the nondominant hand, between the index or middle finger (placed in the mouth) and the thumb on the skin surface outside the mouth, beneath the mandible. In that way, one individual can perform the entire procedure, the dominant hand being free for the syringe holder.

Nodes in the axilla or the supraclavicular fossa may lie very close to the pleural surface, so that some thought should be given to avoiding a possible pneumothorax. This problem was discussed in the section on potential complications of breast aspiration.

Nodes in the axilla can be very difficult to puncture accurately until after gaining considerable experience in this procedure. They are often very mobile. If located high in the axilla, they must be pulled downward by the examining fingertips and then stabilized by pressing the nodes against the lateral chest wall. Palpation is facilitated by having the muscles that border the axilla in relaxation. We find that these goals are facilitated by sitting beside the seated patient and asking the patient to rest his or her hand on the physician's shoulder. As noted previously, however, for nonrecumbent patients, it is important to ensure that should the patient be weak or should fainting occur, no fall or injury ensues. Thus, when executing this maneuver, we generally have an assistant positioned to help support the patient should this become necessary.

### Diagnostic Considerations in Lymph-Node Cytology

The diagnoses that can be made on lymph-node aspirations fall into broad categories, including benign lymphoid tissue, infectious processes, metastatic neoplasms, and malignant lymphoma. The relative frequency with which these groups are studied depends very much on the patient population in a given practice.

*Reactive Lymph Nodes*    Benign, hyperplastic lymph nodes are very common. These often present in clinical situations where the possibility of malignancy seems remote. When persistent, they can be clinically troublesome.

The cytologic hallmark of such cases is a pattern of heterogeneity among the aspirated cells. That is, large lymphocytes, small lymphocytes, macrophages, neutrophils, and occasional plasma cells are present. When a good specimen is

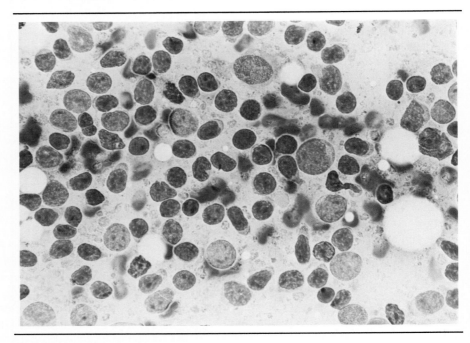

Figure 2.13.
*This well prepared smear from a benign hyperplastic lymph node shows a pattern of heterogeneity, with small lymphocytes and large transformed-appearing lymphocytes. This heterogeneity is indicative of a benign, reactive process (modified Diff-Quik® stain, ×500 before a 34% reduction).*

obtained and the smears are properly prepared, this pattern is readily apparent (Figure 2.13). The etiology of such localized nodal hyperplasia is often clinically undetermined. The expected clinical outcome is resolution. When adenopathy persists, progresses, or spreads to other node groups, repeat aspiration with ICC analysis is indicated.

*Infectious and Granulomatous Lymphadenopathy*    Infectious lymphadenopathy is also commonly aspirated. Layfield et al. describe a protocol for culture of aspirated lymph-node materials.[45] Their criteria for initiating cultures are summarized in Table 2.8. When suspected instances of contamination were excluded, microorganisms were recovered from 21 percent of 44 cases and included bacteria, fungi, and mycobacteria. This yield of infectious organisms is comparable to that obtained by culture of surgically excised lymph nodes.[46] Six unsuspected malignancies were also diagnosed. We agree with these authors that a complete evaluation requires culture for fungi, mycobacteria, and anaerobic organisms, in addition to routine aerobic bacterial cultures. The use of special stains for a rapid evaluation is sometimes rewarding.

It is our practice to perform a separate aspiration and dedicate its entire yield to microbiologic evaluation. Transport media may vary with different types of potential organisms. We consult the microbiology laboratory before obtaining material for culture.

Table 2.8
*Clinical criteria for initiating microbiological culture of material aspirated from lymph nodes*

Fever
Erythema
Pain
Local heat
Purulent-appearing aspiration
Low suspicion of malignancy
Other clinical indications

*Note.* Lymph-node culture protocol developed by Layfield et al.[45]

We have had experience with aspiration of *Mycobacterium tuberculosis* on several occasions. Smears usually show necrotic debris. Giant cells and granulomas are also seen (Figure 2.14). While not completely diagnostic, this pattern is sufficiently suggestive to warrant initiation of culture. If the diagnosis has not been suspected until after the smears are examined, a repeat aspiration can easily be performed for culture. It is our practice in such instances to make an extra air-dried smear. This can be stained with the Auromine-Rhodomine method. Fluorescence microscopy may show mycobacteria. This type of stain is technically more simple than traditional stains for acid-fast bacilli, and it is much easier to screen for the presence of occasional organisms. The necrotic appearance just

Figure 2.14.
*Aspiration smear from a tuberculous lymph node. There is a background of necrosis and a single multinucleated giant cell is seen (modified Diff-Quik® stain, ×160 before a 26% reduction).*

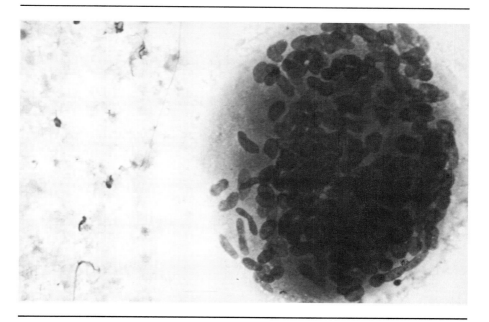

described differs considerably from the cohesive, epithelioid granulomas in a clear background that characterize the cytology of sarcoidosis (Figure 2.15).

Evaluation of potentially infectious or neoplastic lymphadenopathy in patients with the acquired immunodeficiency syndrome (AIDS) is currently of considerable interest. Bottles et al. describe their results with outpatient study of 121 lymph-node aspirations in 113 AIDS patients.[47] Their diagnostic results are summarized in Table 2.9. A majority of their cases showed either hyperplasia or an infectious process. Five malignancies were undiagnosed by initial FNA. The greatest problem was with Hodgkin's disease, in which only one of four histologically diagnosed cases were identified cytologically.

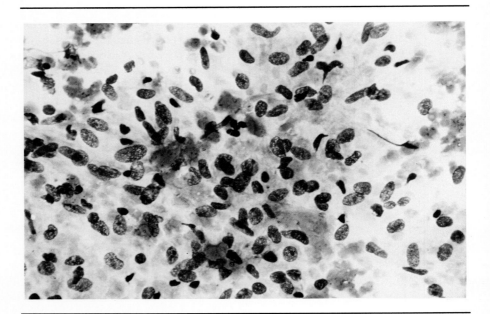

Figure 2.15.
*This cohesive granuloma composed of epithelioid histiocytes is from granulomatous lymphadenitis in sarcoidosis. The clear background is very different from that seen in tuberculous nodes (modified Diff-Quik® stain, ×160 before a 24% reduction).*

Table 2.9
*Diagnostic results in 121 lymph-node aspirations from 113 AIDS patients*

| | | |
|---|---|---|
| Lymphoid hyperplasia | 50% | (*n* = 60) |
| Non-Hodgkin's malignant lymphoma | 20% | (*n* = 24) |
| Mycobacterial infection | 17% | (*n* = 21) |
| Kaposi's sarcoma | 10% | (*n* = 12) |
| Hodgkin's disease | | 1 case |
| Carcinoma | | 3 cases |

Data are from Bottles et al.[47]

We have previously reported three cases of atypical mycobacterial infections in AIDS patients and noted a distinctive appearance of aspirated histiocytes on air-dried, Romanowsky-stained smears.[48] In such preparations, the affected histiocytes showed numerous clear (negatively stained), cylindrical cytoplasmic rods (Figure 2.16). Acid-fast stains showed acid-fast bacilli that were shown by culture to be atypical mycobacteria. When present, this finding is characteristic of these infections. It appears to be unique to AIDS patients, who harbor a very large burden of organisms.

*Metastatic Malignancies*   The most commonly diagnosed malignancies in lymph-node cytology are metastases from other primary sites. These may have been previously diagnosed so that nodal disease represents progression of the tumor; they may be the first indication of malignancy; or they may be diagnosed at the same time as the primary tumor. In the third instance, this staging information often severely circumscribes the patient's therapeutic options. That such information can be rapidly and inexpensively obtained with great accuracy is one of the most useful and often humane applications of FNA. In this way, many patients are spared unnecessary delays and painful surgical procedures that offer little or no benefit and may be very costly.

It is often possible to identify a metastatic malignancy as adenocarcinoma, squamous-cell carcinoma, small-cell carcinoma, malignant melanoma, or a

Figure 2.16.
*Lymph-node aspiration from an AIDS patient infected with atypical mycobacteria. The organisms are seen here as clear cytoplasmic cylinders in an affected histiocyte (modified Diff-Quik® stain, ×1000 before a 34% reduction).*

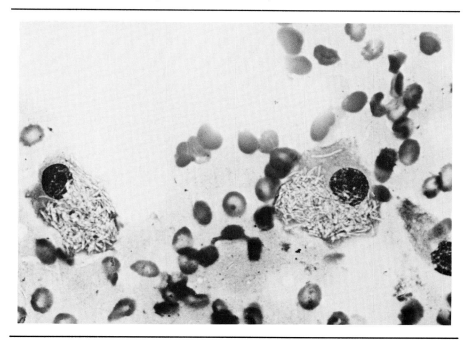

germ-cell tumor by cytologic study. Determinations of primary site may be much more difficult or completely impossible. Clinical and radiographic studies, when combined with the cytologic diagnosis, will often narrow the range of diagnostic possibilities considerably to a few likely choices. Once again, FNA is a first-line or primary care method that can direct further evaluation along specific lines.

Even in the face of metastatic disease, these fundamental pathologic distinctions often have significance. Squamous-cell malignancies may be amenable to radiation therapy, while many germ-cell tumors or small-cell anaplastic (oat cell) carcinomas can be chemically treated. The patient with advanced adenocarcinoma or malignant melanoma may have very few therapeutic options. Furthermore, it is adenocarcinoma and malignant melanoma for which primary sites most commonly remain occult even after extensive investigation.

The cytologic identification of metastatic disease is often very straightforward. The cells have been described as "alien" by Soderstrom,[12] and they stand out against the lymphoid elements that are similar to those in Figure 2.13. In most series, the diagnostic yield of metastatic malignancy in lymph-node aspiration exceeds 90 percent and often approaches 100 percent.[2,12,49–55] These results are comparable to those achieved by surgical excision of the node. Typical examples of squamous-cell carcinoma, adenocarcinoma, malignant melanoma, and a malignant germ-cell tumor of testicular origin are shown in Figures 2.17 through 2.20, respectively.

Figure 2.17.
*Metastatic squamous-cell carcinoma of the larynx, aspirated from a cervical lymph node. The malignant cells show dense orange cytoplasm, with sharp borders indicative of keratin production. Such smears frequently show background inflammation and necrosis (Papanicolaou stain, X250 before a 26% reduction).*

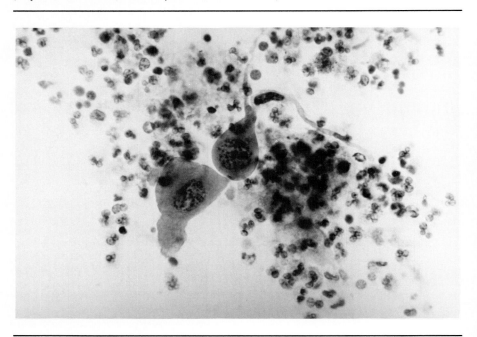

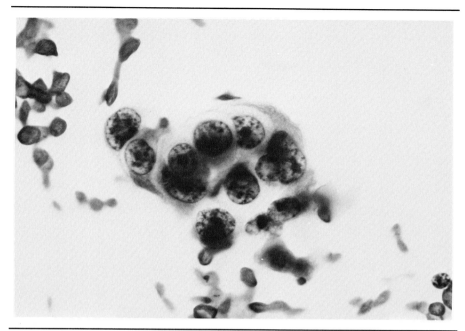

Figure 2.18.
*Metastatic pulmonary adenocarcinoma aspirated from a supraclavicular lymph node. The cells show traditional nuclear features of malignancy and have clear cytoplasm (Papanicolaou stain, ×250 before a 34% reduction).*

When poorly differentiated malignant cells are aspirated from an enlarged lymph node, it may be impossible to determine whether they represent a large-cell malignant lymphoma or a metastatic lesion. This is one of the limitations of routine morphologic investigation of malignant neoplasms and can be a problem in surgical pathology, as well as cytology. In such cases, the precise diagnosis will often be obtained by careful application of special studies, such as ICC stains. Particular specimen handling requirements needed for such studies were discussed in Chapter 1 and are further elaborated in the following section on malignant lymphoma.

*Malignant Lymphoma*   In patients suffering from malignant lymphoma (ML), the potential applications of FNA are several, as summarized in Table 2.10. Of these applications, it is the initial diagnosis of ML by FNA that has aroused the greatest controversy. In the past, some feared that distortion by needle aspiration would compromise the quality of histologic examination if excision was ultimately required for diagnosis. We have found this not to be a problem. As stated by Kline et al., "There is no distortion of nodal architecture when excisional biopsy is necessary for final diagnosis."[49]

The accuracy of diagnosis of ML by FNA has been questioned by some.[56,57] The primary reason for this is the complexity of contemporary classifications of lymphoma. These are based not only on the cytologic characteristics of the

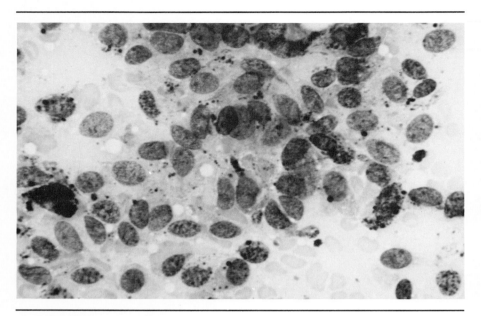

Figure 2.19.
*Metastatic malignant melanoma aspirated from an inguinal lymph node. The cells are uniform, often spindled, and have abundant dark melanin pigment granules (modified Diff-Quik® stain, ×250 before a 26% reduction). (Photograph courtesy of Dr. Charles A. Horwitz, Metropolitan–Mt. Sinai Hospital, Minneapolis, Minnesota.)*

malignant cells, but also on nodal architecture, as assessed with histologic sections, and on immunophenotypic analysis based on staining patterns with panels of monoclonal antibodies.

The details of cytologic diagnosis of ML and the classification of this group of disorders are beyond the scope of this book. In general, a monotonous (homogeneous) population of cells contrasts sharply with the pattern of heterogeneity typical of benign processes. Examples of common malignant lymphomas of low and high grade are shown in Figures 2.21 and 2.22, respectively. These should be compared with the benign lymphoid tissue depicted in Figure 2.13. Mixed cell lymphomas are cytologically heterogenous and are more difficult to recognize; a confident diagnosis usually requires immunophenotypic marker studies.

Immunophenotypic markers can be evaluated in FNA material.[58,59] When combined with cytologic findings, this type of analysis allows accurate diagnosis of high-grade lymphomas. Tissue architecture (nodular vs. diffuse) must be assessed in some low-grade lymphomas of B-cell origin, but in the high-grade types, FNA has the potential to replace histopathology as the primary diagnostic method.

Marker analysis is best performed on cells suspended in phosphate-buffered saline at the time of FNA. These are then applied to glass slides by the cytocentrifuge.[58] In Sweden, we have seen cases in which diagnosis by FNA,

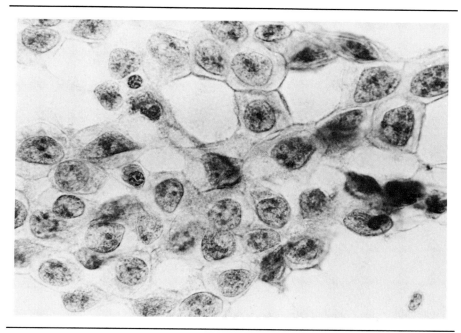

Figure 2.20.
*This retroperitoneal lymph node aspirate was obtained with radiologic guidance. The smears showed large tumor cells with abundant, clear cytoplasm. In this case, the seminoma was primary in the testis (Papanicolaou stain, ×788 before a 34% reduction).*

Table 2.10
*Applications of aspiration cytology to patients with malignant lymphoma*

Initial diagnosis
Staging
Confirmation of recurrence
Diagnosis of second malignancy
Diagnosis of infection
Diagnosis of transformation to a more aggressive type of lymphoma

classification by marker analysis, and induction with chemotherapeutic treatment have all taken place within a few hours of the patient's presentation at the clinic.

Recognition or suspicion of lymphoma may be sufficient in the primary-care setting. The patient is then referred for evaluation and treatment at a center able to repeat the FNA and perform the marker studies. Technical excellence and interpretive expertise is required for dependable results, so that smaller facilities that evaluate and treat lymphoma patients only rarely will need to refer these problems to a large oncology institution.

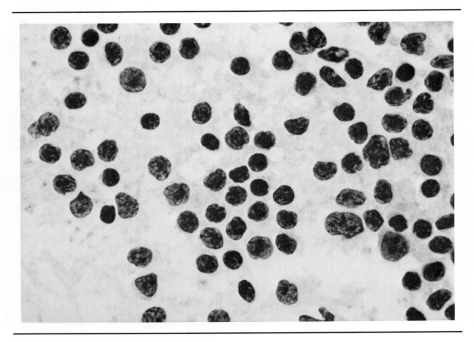

Figure 2.21.
*FNA smear of a low-grade malignant lymphoma. The cells are monomorphous. Their nuclei are larger than those of mature small lymphocytes and are surrounded by very little cytoplasm. Several nuclei show clefts, grooves, or indentations. This would be classified as small cleaved cell malignant lymphoma (poorly differentiated lymphocytic lymphoma) (Papanicolaou stain, ×500 before a 34% reduction).*

*Hodgkin's Disease*   Cytologic diagnosis of Hodgkin's disease requires identification of Reed-Sternberg cells and their variants in an appropriate background of heterogeneous lymphoid tissue. Microscopically, this is analogous to the situation described for diagnosis of metastatic carcinoma. In both conditions, large cellular elements are distinctly out of context in the background of polymorphous (and thus benign-appearing) lymphoid tissue. In Hodgkin's disease, these are single Reed-Sternberg cells that must be sought carefully. The smear pattern in Hodgkin's disease can be mimicked by some T-cell lymphomas or polymorphous B-cell malignancies. Thus, this diagnosis is sometimes less clear-cut than previously thought. In carcinoma, by contrast, clumps of tumor cells may be very obvious even at low magnification. Cohesive clustering of neoplastic elements is not a feature of hematopoietic neoplasms, including Hodgkin's disease.

Any lymph-node aspiration that at first seems to show only heterogeneous, benign-appearing lymphoid tissue should probably be searched for Reed-Sternberg cells. As reviewed previously, some benign cells (especially binucleated macrophages) and several types of nonlymphoid malignant cells may resemble Reed-Sternberg cells.[60] Identification of the diagnostic elements must be based

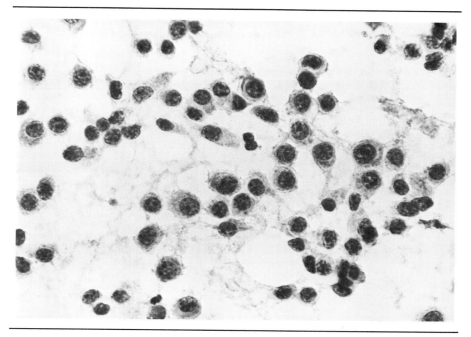

Figure 2.22.
*FNA smear of an immunoblastic malignant lymphoma. These large cells are very monotonous and plasmacytoid in appearance (modified Diff-Quik® stain, ×312 before a 34% reduction).*

on sound morphologic criteria. A typical case of Hodgkin's disease with prominent Reed-Sternberg cells in shown in Figure 2.23.

If present in low numbers, Reed-Sternberg cells may not be sampled by aspiration, or they may be overlooked at the microscope. A false-negative diagnosis then results. This probably accounts for the persistent 5 to 10 percent false-negative rate when series of Hodgkin's disease cases are studied by needle aspiration.[61–63] Another cause for false-negative needle aspiration of Hodgkin's disease is excessive fibrosis and low cellularity. This degree of fibrosis may also cause false-negative aspirations in nodes involved by metastatic carcinoma. This problem is illustrated in Chapter 3.

*Atypical Lymph-Node Aspiration*　Some lymph-node aspirations will be cytologically atypical but not clearly diagnostic of malignant lymphoma. Some diagnostic problems may be resolved by serologic, microbiologic, or follow-up information. Some will require repeat FNA with immunologic marker studies or eventual surgical excision for accurate diagnosis. It is important to remember that mixed-cell lymphomas or T-cell malignancies can present this cytologic picture. Acute Epstein-Barr virus infection (infectious mononucleosis) can cause striking lymphadenopathy that may clinically and cytologically suggest malignant lymphoma.[60] Serologic studies are usually diagnostic.

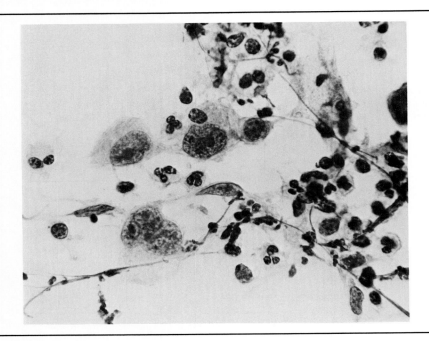

Figure 2.23.
*This typical example of Hodgkin's disease studied by FNA shows Reed-Sternberg cells in a background of polymorphous lymphoid tissue (Papanicolaou stain, ×800 before a 34% reduction).*

## Aspiration of Salivary Glands

Technical aspects of parotid-gland FNA are not significantly different from those of other subcutaneous masses, such as lymph nodes. All but the largest submandibular masses may require bimanual palpation for localization and aspiration. This was described in our consideration of submandibular lymph nodes. Intraoral masses that are covered by a smooth mucosa are frequently derived from minor salivary glands. Such lesions can occur in any part of the oral tissues and may be aspirated much as one would study subcutaneous masses. Topical anesthesia in the form of a spray can be easily applied to the mucosa.

The majority of salivary-gland masses are cysts, hyperplastic intraparotid lymph nodes, other inflammatory lesions, benign mixed tumors (pleomorphic adenoma), monomorphic adenomas (Warthin's tumor constitutes the majority of lesions in this category), adenoid cystic carcinoma or low-grade mucoepidermoid carcinoma. Most of these can be readily diagnosed by FNA. High-grade carcinomas (which may be very difficult to subclassify reproducibly), primary malignant lymphoma, and other malignancies are uncommon; most are readily recognized as malignant in cytologic preparations.

Salivary-gland tumors are histologically quite diverse. Some entities are uncommon, and some are not well documented in the FNA literature. Thus, problems in microscopic interpretation will occur from time to time and will necessitate surgical excision.[9] This does not detract from the fact that most masses represent one of the aforementioned relatively common entities and are readily diagnosed by FNA.

Considering this differential diagnosis, it may be difficult to stratify clinically the patients who have no presenting problem except a salivary gland mass. It is noteworthy, however, that most cases of parotid masses associated with pain or evidence of facial-nerve damage are malignant.

These issues, however, do not constitute the greatest impediment to implementation of salivary-gland FNA. Fear of complications and a feeling that the information obtained by FNA will not alter patient management prevent many from applying this valuable method to patients with salivary-gland masses.

Fear of complications, which at first seems well founded, is seen to be unreasonable when the literature on this subject is carefully assessed. The facial nerve and its radicals divide within and course through the substance of the parotid gland. Some fear damage to this nerve either directly by the needle or as a result of compression by an enlarging hematoma. While such a fear may be reasonable if one is using large, cutting-type core biopsy instruments, no instance of such damage has been reported by those using 25- or 23-gauge ("fine") needles. The only local complication of salivary-gland FNA seems to be the formation of small hematomas,[64] but even this is not noted in most series.[2,65]

The other complication feared by some clinicians is local tumor recurrence. This is based on the fact that the most common salivary-gland neoplasm is the benign mixed tumor (pleomorphic adenoma). Metastasizing cases of histologically benign mixed tumor are reportably rare. The real danger with this tumor is that if surgically violated by incision or by a large cutting needle, it has a strong tendency to be followed by multifocal local recurrence or implantation. Such recurrences may be very difficult to control. Fearing this outcome and noting that benign mixed tumor is very common, some practitioners forego all salivary-gland aspiration. In fact, when small needles are used, there is no reported incident of such recurrence after FNA.[66,67]

We agree with Cohen et al., who summarize the literature by noting, "there have been no reports of infection, nerve damage, needle tract contamination or dissemination of tumor cells resulting in distant metastases."[68] It cannot be overemphasized that the small size of the needles used for aspiration is the key to making this a safe procedure. Given that much of this work is now 20 or more years old and involves large series of carefully studied patients reported by highly authoritative physicians, it is surprising that some clinicians are still citing fear of nerve damage and tumor recurrence as reasons not to use salivary-gland FNA.

The remaining impediment to implementation of salivary gland FNA is the feeling that it will have little effect on patient management. The train of thought leading to this conclusion is something like the following: (1) Malignant salivary-gland masses that have neither clinical nor radiographic features of malignancy are not common. (2) Cytopathologists could diagnose benign mixed tumor in every case and be correct 80 percent of the time without even looking at the smears because this tumor accounts for most salivary-gland neoplasms. (3) There is only one surgical approach to benign or low-grade malignant masses of the parotid; this involves complete removal with a surrounding margin of normal tissue.

Qizilbash and Young describe their progression over time from the aforementioned point of view to cautious aspiration of selected cases. As applications expanded, the authors "were pleasantly surprised at the usefulness of needle aspiration biopsy for salivary gland swellings."[69] Ultimately, recognizing that complications were very rare and that the nature of clinically ambiguous lesions could be clarified by FNA, they began to apply FNA to virtually all salivary-gland masses. Furthermore, these authors noted that "some patients in whom the diagnosis seemed most obvious were those in whom needle aspiration provided a diagnosis that differed most radically from the presumed diagnosis suspected by the clinician." We agree completely with these authors' conclusion when they "recommend routine needle aspiration of all salivary gland lesions no matter how obvious the diagnosis appears when the patient first presents."

## Fine-Needle Aspiration of Skin Nodules

Any palpable nodule can be aspirated. In North America, however, the tendency is to use punch biopsy or excisional biopsy of cutaneous masses. If a malignancy (other than basal-cell carcinoma) is strongly suspected on clinical grounds, some will proceed at once to complete excision rather than use any type of biopsy.

While the range of dermal lesions that can be aspirated on rare occasions is extremely broad, two are commonly studied: keratinous cyst and dermal recurrence of breast carcinoma. The first of these is the *keratinous cyst*, also known as epidermal inclusion cyst or sebaceous cyst. These firm, subcutaneous, dome-shaped dermal nodules may be up to several cm in greatest dimension. Their nature is usually suspected by the experienced surgeon. Patients with a history of malignancy may be referred for evaluation of suspected metastatic disease. The thick, white, caseous content of squamous debris is immediately apparent when expelled from the needle. Also, the characteristic rotten egg odor of this material is far from subtle. Thus, a diagnosis can often be rendered at the bedside before microscopic examination. In the clinical setting of known cancer, this finding can be very reassuring. The rapidity with which this finding is discovered is always welcome. An example of this situation is offered in Chapter 3.

Dermal recurrence of breast carcinoma is another setting in which cutaneous FNA can be very useful in providing rapid, reliable information by very inexpensive means. Such lesions usually take the form of small (<5 mm), round or oval, firm, pale nodules. They may be much more apparent as the examining fingertips are moved lightly over the skin surface than they initially seem to be on visual inspection. Needles of 25 (0.5 mm) gauge are very suitable for aspiration of such nodules. The 5/8-inch (16 mm) length is best.

If one attempts aspiration of these tiny subcutaneous nodules by going directly through the overlying skin, the needle will often be moved above the skin surface as the aspiration proceeds. When this happens, suction will be lost, and the quantity of material removed may be small. An alternative approach is shown in Figures 2.24 and 2.25. First, using the internally sterile plastic cap in which the needle is packaged, the needle is bent to a 45° angle after the cap is loosened (see Figure 2.24). As shown in Figure 2.25, the needle enters the skin at a small distance from the nodule. The nodule is then punctured from its deep surface, and the oscillating motion of FNA is carried out. The skin will usually be elevated or

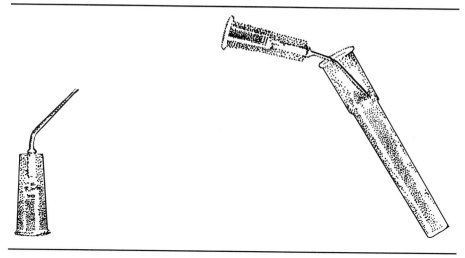

Figure 2.24.
*The needle hub is held in one hand, while the other loosens the plastic cap. Before the cap is completely removed, it is used to bend the needle to an angle of approximately 45°. The point of needle insertion into the hub is used as the fulcrum against which the needle-cap-lever turns.*

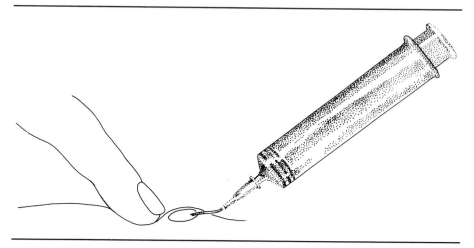

Figure 2.25.
*The examiner's fingertip is placed near the small dermal nodule. When pressure is applied, the nodule will often protrude slightly and be less mobile. The tip of the bent needle (Figure 2.24) enters the skin at a point several millimeters from the nodule to be punctured. The nodule is then punctured from its deep surface.*

tented when the needle is within the dermal nodule. In this way, the location of the needle tip can be monitored, and penetration of the overlying skin—with resultant loss of suction—will not occur. When aspirated in this manner, even tiny dermal nodules of recurrent breast carcinoma often yield highly cellular smears that are clearly diagnostic of recurrent malignancy. Alternatively, the Zajdela technique can be used (see Chapter 1).

Larger dermal recurrences or metastases can be approached as with any palpable mass. FNA offers a rapid, accurate means of diagnosing such lesions.

## Palpable Masses of the Abdomen and Retroperitoneum

In Sweden, many masses in the abdomen and retroperitoneum are studied initially by FNA. In North America, however, it is very uncommon to see such patients before radiographic study (ultrasound or CT scan) has localized the lesion and its potential extensions or metastases. Such studies will often limit considerably the differential diagnostic possibilities that the cytopathologist must consider. It is also the case that such lesions are usually aspirated by the radiologist with radiographic or ultrasonographic guidance, to ensure accurate needle placement.

When masses are readily palpable, however, there is little contraindication to direct transcutaneous FNA at the bedside. Physicians familiar with the advantages of FNA may send the patient for this study prior to radiographic evaluation. When the CT scan is available, confidence in the patient's safety is often very great indeed. We have used this approach for study of the palpably enlarged liver, which by CT scan shows a large burden of metastatic tumor. Such "blind" aspirations without radiographic guidance are frequently diagnostic and spare the patient other costly, painful studies. The liver can be localized by palpation and percussion. Furthermore, with the CT image in hand, it is possible to be certain that no lung tissue overlies the selected area of aspiration. Longer needles than those often used may be required. We begin with the 25-gauge (0.5 mm) needle of 2-inch (5 cm) length. If this is not sufficient, we proceed to a 3 1/2-inch (8.8 cm) spinal needle. An example of such a case can be found in Chapter 3 (Case 6).

Most palpable abdominal or retroperitoneal masses can be safely aspirated. A particular issue relates to the aspiration of ovarian masses. Diagnostic needle aspiration of the ovary has been used extensively in several European centers[70–72] but has not been widely accepted in North America and Britain.[9,73–76] Without examining the data that underlie these contrasting points of view, Table 2.11 summarizes some of the published reasons given by several authors for their unwillingness to embrace this method.

We add our support to that of Koss et al.[77] for the suggested indications for ovarian aspiration advanced by Geier and Strecker.[73] These are limited to the following: "(1) recurrence of a previously diagnosed and treated ovarian cancer, (2) rare cases of poor physical condition of patients that do not allow laparotomy and (3) in benign cysts, the possible derivation of some additional information by measurement of the unconjugated estradiol-17." These comments also apply to transrectal or transvaginal aspiration of the ovary. Thus, one contribution made by preaspiration radiographic evaluation is determination of the mass's organ of origin.

Some fear the consequences of entering the stomach, small intestine, or colon if abdominal aspiration is performed without radiographic guidance in needle

Table 2.11
*Published objections to diagnosis of ovarian masses by needle aspiration*[73-76]

1.  Aspiration may transform a potentially curable tumor into an incurable one by tumor spillage. This makes aspiration a high-risk procedure with little justification.

2.  It is difficult to distinguish borderline tumors from malignant neoplasms by cytology alone.

3.  Ovarian tumors are histologically very diverse and frequently cannot be reliably subclassified in cytologic preparations.

4.  Proper treatment requires precise knowledge of tumor type and stage, which can only be obtained surgically.

5.  Aspiration is often a redundant and unnecessary procedure because excision is usually required for proper management.

6.  There is a 1.6% incidence of postaspiration pelvic infections following transvaginal or transrectal aspiration ($N = 191$ palpable ovarian masses).

placement. In fact, penetration of bowel loops is quite common when radiologists direct needles into deep-seated lesions such as those in the pancreas. In one study of 2500 transabdominal and transthoracic FNAs from Toronto General Hospital, the authors cite no instance of an infectious or hemorrhagic complication of bowel penetration.[8] They emphasize that the needles used for these studies are smaller than surgical suture material, which is commonly placed in the bowel wall with impunity.

By far the most striking evidence that penetration of the bowel by fine needles is without infectious complications comes from large series of transrectal prostatic aspirations. These are discussed in the following subsection.

## Prostate Aspirations

The methods described herein can be applied to transrectal or transvaginal aspiration of palpable pelvic masses of different types. The previous reflections on ovarian aspiration are applicable, as many of these are aspirated by a transvaginal approach.

The prostate is first examined by digital rectal palpation in the usual fashion. The location, size, and texture of masses is noted and compared with those described by the referring physician. Patients referred by urologists may be much more highly selected than those referred by internists or general practitioners and will more frequently have distinct, localized nodules suitable for aspiration. Considerable practice is required to gain proficiency in digital examination of the prostate. This skill is essential and must be well developed prior to attempting prostatic aspirations.

Both this examination and the aspiration can be accomplished either with the patient in lithotomy position (see Figure 2.27) or standing. We prefer the former. It is convenient for the physician and comfortable for the patients, most of whom are elderly. The rare individual who faints (or as in one case we have observed, experiences angina pectoris) is thus in no danger of injury from a fall.

The needle used for prostatic aspiration is 22 gauge (0.7 mm) and 20 cm (7 7/8 inch) in length. It is guided to the palpable lesion by following the index finger of the nondominant hand as it is placed on the mass. This is accomplished by means of a needle guide devised by Franzen (Figure 2.26). Distally, this features a ring that fits over the tip of the index finger. This is sometimes open along one edge so that the ring can be expanded or collapsed to fit fingers of various sizes. The ring is mounted to a long, thin, tubular needle guide that reaches to the palm of the examiner's hand. The proximal end of this tube has a trumpet-bell-like flare to facilitate entry of the long needle. The needle guide's final feature is a small flat plate near its center. This is attached by a thumb screw that can be loosened, allowing the plate to be moved along the length of the needle guide tube. During the procedure, this appropriately positioned plate is held firmly in the palm of the nondominant hand by the second and third fingers. This provides great stability to the positioning of the needle guide.

Once the needle guide is installed on the physician's gloved nondominant hand, its tip is covered by a rubber finger cot. (A finger cut from an extra latex glove can be substituted, if necessary.) This prevents filling of the needle guide with fecal material and mucus as it is placed in the rectum and brought to rest pressing on the previously localized mass. This simple and inexpensive step is essential and greatly improves specimen quality.

When this assembly (hand, glove, needle guide, and finger cot) is ready, a water-soluble lubricant is applied and the index finger is introduced rectally and

Figure 2.26.
*The Franzen needle guide for prostatic aspiration is shown here on the physician's gloved left hand. Its components are described in the text. A finger cot is in place. (Photograph courtesy of Dr. Charles A. Horwitz, Metropolitan–Mt. Sinai Hospital, Minneapolis, Minnesota.)*

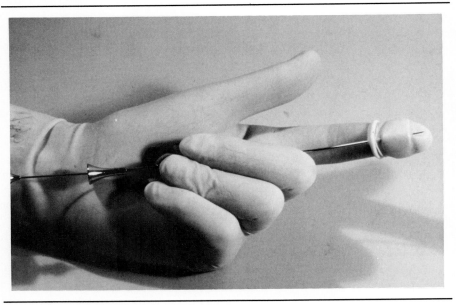

brought to rest on the mass. It is apparent that the needle's exit will be from the end of the guide tube, which lies along the palmar surface of the index finger. Because we generally palpate nodules with the exact tip of the finger, the needle will traverse the rectal mucosa and enter the prostate 0.5 to 1.0 cm closer to the anus than the point being localized. When small nodules are under study, the fingertip must be moved proximally along the rectal mucosa by this distance, to ensure accurate puncture of the target.

At this point, the needle is now taken up. It already will have been attached to a syringe, which is itself held by the syringe pistol. The ease with which it can be introduced into the flare of the needle guide compensates for the unwieldy nature of this long needle. As the needle is slowly advanced in the needle guide, a mark near its hub approaches the needle-guide opening. When this is at the level of the entry to the trumpet-bell-like opening, the needle tip will be located at the needle guide's exit and is thus poised to enter the rectal mucosa. At this point, the neophyte will fear sticking his or her fingertip. Because the needle exits the needle guide below the fingertip and is aimed straight ahead, this does not happen and has never been described by those schooled in the use of this device.

The needle can now be advanced into the prostate itself. A distance of 1 to 2 cm is sufficient. This distance can be judged by watching the needle progress further into the needle guide opening, which is furnished with markings at 1-cm intervals. A low amplitude in-and-out motion similar to that used for percutaneous aspiration is then executed for 5 to 10 seconds.

Figure 2.27 shows one of the authors in the act of prostatic aspiration. In

Figure 2.27.
*Prostatic fine needle aspiration. The patient is in the lithotomy position. The left hand index finger, bearing the needle guide is placed in the rectum (see text for description). The syringe pistol is held in the right hand. The physician's foot rests on a small step-stool (not shown), so that his knee provides a stable support for the hand that bears the needle guide.*

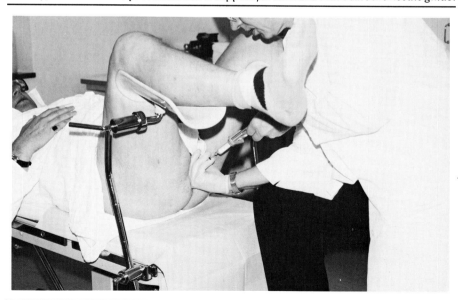

addition to the techniques just described, note that the physician's knee is raised and supports the forearm. This is helpful in keeping the nondominant hand and its needle guide very still and secure. This is accomplished by means of placing a small one-step stool at the foot of the examining table. This stool also makes it easier for older patients to get up onto the examining table in clinics where it cannot be lowered sufficiently.

When the aspiration is completed, the needle is withdrawn, and the nondominant hand's index finger is removed from the rectum. The material in the needle is expressed onto a glass slide, and smears are prepared as discussed in Chapter 1. Malignancies often yield a semisolid droplet, while aspirations of benign glands are associated with copious fluid. Thus, optimal handling requires some flexibility in the technique of smear preparation.

Only the nondominant hand's index finger is contaminated with fecal material. Experienced practitioners find it convenient to manipulate the needle and slides using the thumb with the ring and middle fingers of the still-gloved nondominant hand. In this way, the glove, needle guide, finger cot, and lubricant are left in place. This means that multiple aspirations can be accomplished without the delay involved in refitting these appliances. In this fashion, two to three aspirations can be completed and smears prepared in 2 minutes or less. Alternatively, an assistant can prepare the smears while the operator begins the next aspiration.

Prostate FNA is clearly more complex than usual percutaneous procedures. The target is not visualized, and a mental image of relationships among the lesion, the fingertip, and the distal opening of the needle guide must be maintained. Considerable practice is needed to acquire and maintain skills in this area.

### Infections Resulting from Prostate Aspiration

Infections are virtually unheard-of when palpable lesions are aspirated through the skin. If infections were ever a problem in FNA, certainly this would become apparent in transrectal prostatic aspiration. It is not uncommon to see rectal mucosa, prostatic tissue, and small amounts of stool in a single smear, indicating the great potential for contamination of tissues with infectious material. As noted previously, infectious problems are very rare when bowel loops are penetrated by the needle during FNA of abdominal or retroperitoneal masses.[8]

Transient febrile reactions were noted in 1 percent of 508 prostatic aspirations, and the extremely serious complication of Gram-negative sepsis was seen in four of 14,000 cases.[78,79] Thus, infections are extremely uncommon in these patients, especially when FNA is compared with other means for obtaining tissue from the prostate. Preaspiration antibiotic prophylaxis was not used in those patients who had neither valvular heart disease nor a cardiovascular prosthesis. An increased risk of infection has been noted if seminal-vesicle material is identified during microscopic examination of the smears. It is our practice to give a brief course of antibiotics when this occurs.

### Current Trends in Diagnosis of Prostate Lesions

In North America, there has recently been a marked trend away from the use of FNA as a diagnostic method for prostatic nodules. Most urologists are accustomed to performing core biopsies for diagnosis of prostatic nodules, and histopathologists are comfortable interpreting the material obtained. Problems with this approach include the need to perform the procedure in the operating room, frequent complications, and a significant false negative rate in the diagnosis of carcinoma (reviewed by Stanley et al.[80]).

Use of FNA was in part increased by the fact that it is a low-cost office procedure that has few risks, requires no anesthesia, and has an acceptable false-negative rate in experienced hands. Its widespread use was inhibited by the lack of training many urologists have in this method and the fact that many pathologists cannot confidently interpret the material obtained. Furthermore, there persists the mistaken notion (discussed in our introduction to this volume) that FNA is somehow inherently inferior to tissue biopsy and produces very small specimens.

Thus, the introduction of small (21 gauge) core biopsy instruments into clinical urology has been welcomed. Urologists are comfortable with this technique, and pathologists feel confident in seeing tissue sections (albeit very small ones). Because this needle can be used in the office without complications or anesthesia, many of the factors that might have motivated the wider use of FNA are no longer operative. Furthermore, it gives a core of tissue welcomed by all pathologists. Its use with or without ultrasound guidance has given good results.[81,82]

The histopathologists' preference for section material versus the cytopathologists' comfort with smear material is largely one of training and experience; prostatic carcinoma can be readily diagnosed with either type of specimen. The most important diagnostic possibilities for a prostatic nodule are benign hyperplasia versus adenocarcinoma. The distinction is based on the morphology of the epithelial (glandular) cells. A core of tissue (even a 21-gauge core) is fairly impressive visually. In fact, however, it often consists largely of stroma and may contain only a small percentage of epithelium on which a diagnosis is based. FNA, on the other hand, concentrates the epithelium and extracts little or no stroma. Furthermore, the volume of tissue traversed by the needle is much greater for FNA than for core biopsy. The result is that FNA often provides a greater quantity of diagnostic tissue than does a core biopsy.

Only clinicians skillful at prostatic aspiration working in concert with cytopathologists experienced in the interpretation of smears will be able to determine the relative merits of FNA and small-gauge core biopsy. Based on currently available data, we agree with Kaye and Horwitz that "its [small gauge biopsy] exact role in relation to FNA cytology needs to be determined."[82] We suggest that if the methods are compared by individuals skillful in execution and interpretation of both, the improved sampling of the diagnostically significant epithelium by FNA will show this method to be superior. On the other hand, if performance of prostatic aspiration and interpretation of smear material continue to be uncommon skills, small-gauge core biopsy may ultimately be the preferred method.

## REPORTING OF RESULTS IN FINE-NEEDLE ASPIRATION

This discussion is aimed primarily at pathologists who must report their findings in a concise but complete manner and must bear in mind particular medicolegal issues. The complete reporting method we describe is for use by those who both perform the aspiration and interpret the microscopic findings. Those performing only part of this task will issue only portions of such a report.

## Medicolegal Considerations in the Reporting of Results

In the section on breast FNA, we discussed potential malpractice issues that stem from the inevitable, small, but irreducible false-negative rate of FNA, as it is applied to the very large number of patients with apparently benign breast disease. It is a very important principle of risk management that accurate documentation of the physician's actions provides the best defense during litigation. The FNA report is the primary means of accomplishing this goal.

Potential problems arising from FNA are summarized in Table 2.12. These can be categorized as false-positive diagnoses of malignancy, false-negative diagnoses of malignancy, and complications of the procedure. Many writers and practitioners direct their energy to avoiding the potential complications of FNA. Most of these are extremely rare when thin needles are used by well-educated, experienced physicians. We have briefly discussed some of these issues in relation to FNA of particular body sites (breast, salivary glands, prostate). Our emphasis has been the rarity of these problems. The greatest source of liability arises not from patients injured by the procedure but from the diagnoses that are rendered.

False-positive diagnoses of malignancy are very uncommon, and virtually always occur at the microscope. These are beyond the scope of this book. False-negative diagnoses of malignancy, however, represent the major source of potential liability for the FNA physician. Microscopy is one origin of this type of error. Table 2.12 lists several other causes of false-negative diagnoses. Most of this book is actually directed to minimizing these errors by application of optimal techniques at each step of the FNA process. As noted earlier, we feel that more problems in FNA diagnosis occur at the bedside than at the microscope.

Table 2.12
*Types of problems for which the FNA physician may incur medicolegal liability*

| False-Negative Diagnoses of Malignancy | False-Positive Diagnoses of Malignancy | Complications of the FNA Procedure* |
|---|---|---|
| Inaccurate diagnosis[†] | Inaccurate diagnosis[†,‡] | Pneumothorax |
| Inadequate sampling | | Hematoma |
| Material poorly prepared | | Nerve damage |
| Wrong area aspirated | | Needle tract seeding |
| Intrinsic tumor characteristics | | Tumor dissemination infection |

*All are very rare. Specific problems are discussed in sections on the breast (pneumothorax), salivary gland (hematoma, nerve damage, needle tract seeding, distant metastases), and prostate (infection).

[†]Microscopic interpretation is incorrect.

[‡]Other problems, such as cross-contamination in the laboratory, are issues of laboratory management and quality control. These are beyond the scope of this book.

A final source of liability comes as a surprise to many diagnostic pathologists. Even if a completely accurate interpretation is rendered, failure to communicate this information to the clinician on a timely basis can be a cause for legal action against the pathologist. Kline and Kline have emphasized the need for documentation that verbal or written communication with the clinical team has occurred and that "appropriate communication will defend the practicing cytopathologist against needless litigation."[83]

## Components of the Report

Our reports are modeled on the type of document generally used to report gross, microscopic, and interpretive aspects of surgical biopsy specimens. Clinical, procedural, microscopic, interpretational, and follow-up issues should all be reflected in the final FNA report. This provides a complete assimilation of all available information and adequately documents performance of a high-quality, thorough procedure. Table 2.13 summarizes the components of this type of report. Not every entry will appear in every report.

### Demographics

The demographic section identifies the patient and the referring physician. Note can also be made of other physicians or clinics in need of report copies. Dates should be given for the procedure itself, for specimen receipt in the laboratory, and for report generation. Some reimbursement plans mandate availability of results within a given time span. These dates document the process of specimen preparation and evaluation in the laboratory. Should delays be noted, this information can locate the problem within the laboratory itself or can be used to identify delays in specimen transport to the laboratory or in report generation.

### Patient History

The history section of the report can be brief but should reflect signs, symptoms, chronology, and ancillary studies relevant to the lesion under study. This information is helpful in the cytopathologist's overall assessment of a case. It may highlight the need for additional studies if the cytologic diagnosis does not adequately explain key clinical findings. It also can be used by those conducting reviews of procedures for appropriateness and cost-effectiveness. Finally, it can form an important database for clinical research. It should be documented that the procedure, the cytologic interpretation, and the suggestion of additional studies or follow-up have been conducted in the context of the patient's clinical situation.

### Procedure

The procedure section of the report documents the thoroughness of the aspiration event. Its components describe performance of a procedure tailored to the clinical problem. It permits mention of special handling methods, such as centrifugation of cyst fluid with smears prepared from the cell pellet. Gross findings of diagnostic significance can also be described, such as abundant

Table 2.13
*Components of a complete FNA report*

| | |
|---|---|
| Demographics | Patient name |
| | Age |
| | Sex |
| | Hospital/clinic number |
| | Referring physicians |
| | Laboratory specimen number |
| | Date procedure performed |
| | Date specimen received |
| | Report date |
| History | Location of lesion |
| | Duration of lesion |
| | Size of lesion |
| | Other symptoms (pain, erythema, etc.) |
| | Pertinent laboratory data |
| | Pertinent radiographic findings |
| Procedure | Needle size (gauge) |
| | Number of punctures |
| | Material recovered (amount, appearance) |
| | How much of the palpably abnormal tissue volume was encompassed by the needle's movements within the mass and by overlapping separate punctures? |
| | Special processing (cyst fluids, smears, etc.) |
| Microscopic Finding | Background (necrosis, blood, inflammation, fatty colloid, stroma) |
| | Pertinent negatives (for example, absence of colloid in a thyroid specimen) |
| | Cellular findings |
| | Problems that limit interpretation or classification |
| | Recommendations for additional studies |
| Diagnosis | Site |
| | Diagnosis |
| | "See Description" (directs the reader to special comments, interpretations or suggestions in the microscopic section of the report.) |
| Code | Computer code to permit search of archived reports by aspiration site or diagnosis |

colloid in a thyroid aspiration. If cyst fluid has been aspirated, one should document careful physical examination and reaspiration of any residual mass; not doing so would be construed as incomplete evaluation of a cystic or partially cystic mass.

### Microscopic Finding

Microscopic descriptions should be brief; anyone needing to review these findings will usually examine the glass slides. The key cellular features leading to the final diagnosis should be mentioned. Noncellular findings such as necrosis, inflammation, or thyroid colloid should also be noted.

This descriptive portion of the report is an excellent place for explanatory remarks. (Others place these comments in a separate section under the heading "Comments.") For example, one may identify malignant cells but need to comment on an inability to further classify the neoplasm. Additional studies, recommendations for repeat aspiration, suggestion for surgical biopsy, or follow-up suggestions may be included here. One may also note the need to obtain slides of previous surgical or aspiration specimens, for comparison with the material at hand.

One may also need to express inadequacy of the cytologic diagnosis in the light of clinical findings. The extent to which this is necessary often varies with the expertise of the referring physician. If the physical examination of a breast mass is suspicious for carcinoma, but the cytology shows no malignancy, the surgeon will proceed to surgical biopsy, based on the physical examination. This would be the appropriate response. Others less skilled or experienced in breast examination, and not realizing that FNA has a small false-negative rate (even in such clinically unambiguous cases) may fail to obtain surgical tissue. This would be a serious mismanagement. If the cytopathologist is aware of the clinical findings, further evaluation by surgical means or repeat FNA can be recommended. Similar problems occur in other lesions for which provocative physical findings and false-negative cytology create a dissonance that demands resolution. The cytopathologist is in the unique position of using a detailed knowledge of the procedure's limitations (false-negative rate and difficulties in subclassification of uncommon tumors) to ensure correct application of the cytologic findings.

*Diagnosis*

Our diagnoses are given in two parts: "site" (topography) and "diagnosis" (morphology). To the extent possible, the diagnostic terminology should reflect current practices in surgical pathology. The following are examples:

A. breast, right—fibroadenoma
B. lymph node, cervical, right anterior—metastatic squamous-cell carcinoma
C. parotid gland, left—adenoid cystic carcinoma
D. lymph node, inguinal, left—malignant neoplasm (see description)

When special comments have been made, we follow this type of diagnosis by "(see description)," as shown in the preceding list, example D. The physician is thus directed to consider the cytopathologist's reflections on issues of tumor classification, further evaluation, or patient follow-up.

The historical method of reporting cytologic specimens as inadequate, benign, indeterminate, or malignant is now viewed by most as insufficient. Furthermore, the contemporary cytopathologist is often able to provide diagnoses of much greater specificity. In the uncommon instance in which diagnoses such as D (in the preceding list) are necessary, these should be accompanied by suggestion of means by which the disease process can be more fully classified. (Such classification may or may not be clinically indicated.)

Any attempt to report diagnoses by Papanicolaou's original class system (I through V) or its innumerable modifications is also to be discouraged. (Most workers have abandoned this approach to results reporting, even in gynecologic cytology.)

**UNIVERSITY OF ARKANSAS
FOR MEDICAL SCIENCES**

Name:

Medical Record Number:

Cytology Number:

Sex:

Date of Birth

Age:

**FINE NEEDLE ASPIRATION
CYTOLOGY REPORT**

Clinic:

Doctor:

Date of Service:

Date Received:

## Clinical History

This 32 year old HIV positive male presents with fever of recent onset. Fine needle aspiration of a soft, mobile 2.0 cm right midjugular lymph node is requested. The working clinical diagnosis is "probable malignant lymphoma."

## Procedure

Following alcohol skin preparation, the lymph node was aspirated once with a 25 gauge needle, and four smears were prepared. The needle was moved widely through the palpable abnormality. The patient tolerated the procedure well, with no apparent complications and was instructed to apply pressure to the puncture site with a sterile gauze for five minutes.

After examination of the smears, the aspiration was repeated in the same manner, except that the entire yield was expressed into 5 cc of sterile saline and transported to the mycobacteriology laboratory immediately.

## Microscopic Findings

Smears show numerous histiocytes and occasional lymphocytes. In the air-dried material, negative images of bacilli are present in large numbers. This is indicative of a Mycobacterial infection. Material for culture was submitted, as noted above. (Diagn Cytopathol 6:118-121:1990.) There is no evidence of malignancy.

## Diagnosis

Lymph Node, Cervical-Mycobacterial Infection (Cultures Pending)
(T 08200,E 2000)

Michael W. Stanley, MD                                    Report Date

Figure 2.28.
*Computer generated (and archived) FNA report. See text and Table 2.13 for explanation of its sections.*

Avsändare/svarsmottagare (fullständig adress)

**REMISS, cytologi**

Personnr

Namn

E-sektionen
Radiumhemmet

300120-0000
Patientsson, Patient

| Datum | Rem läkare | Cyt nr |
|---|---|---|
| 930112 | Lundell | |

**AVD FÖR KLINISK CYTOLOGI, Karolinska sjukhuset**

Provtagningsanvisningar, se baksidan

Klinisk diagnos, frågeställning, terapi

Sedan 2 veckor knöl vänster thyreoidealob.
Inga körtlar
Vad är det?

Provet utgörs av/Punktion önskas från

Thyreoidea vänster

Tidigare cytologisk ei histologisk diagnos

Var/nr/år

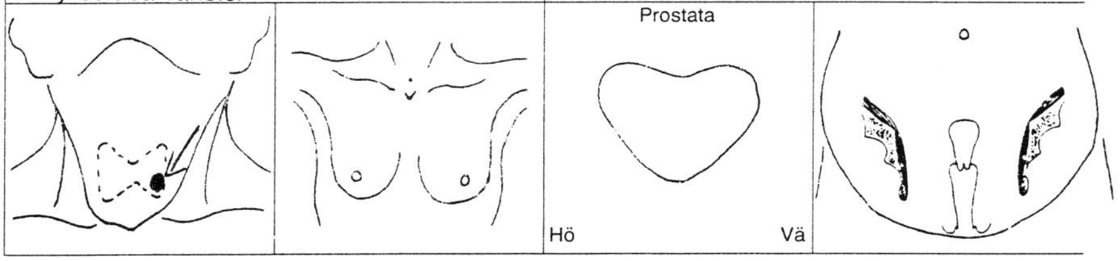

Prostata

Hö　　　　Vä

**CYTOLOGISKT UTLÅTANDE**

Datum

...930112.....

**Thyreoidea, vänster lob**

Solitär, 1-2 cm, rundad, elastisk resistens.
Aspireras några droppar brunfärgad, blodblandad vätska.
Mikroskopi visar kolloid, makrofager  med hemosiderin samt förband av delvis
degenererade follikelceller utan atypi.

**Cytologisk diagnos**
Benign thyreoidenodulus av hyperplasikaraktär med blödningsrester.

Torsten Löwhagen/AT

Adress för provtagning

Avd för Klinisk Cytologi
Radiumhemmet, 1 tr
Karolinska sjukhuset
104 01 STOCKHOLM

Mottagningstider

Mån - Fre 9.00-12.00, 13.30-15.00
Ons 8.00-10.00 (endast prostata)
10.30-12.00 (övriga)

Tfn. tidsbeställning
08-729 43 07

Tfn. provsvar
08-729 43 56

Figure 2.29.
*Swedish FNA report: See text for description of its components.*

*Diagnosis Code*

The report's final component is a computer code for the diagnosis (usually in the SNOMED or SNOP coding system). These consist of both a location code (topography or T code) and a diagnosis code (morphology or M code). Less commonly, an E (etiology) code is used, as in the case of an infectious process. Computerized report archives can be rapidly searched for any of these types of code. Lists can be compiled by site or by diagnosis for use in quality-control activities or research. Most surgical-pathology laboratories in North America already use this type of coding.

*Sample Reports*

Examples of reports from the authors' laboratories are shown in Figures 2.28 and 2.29. The first is a computer-archived verbal report dictated by the cytopathologist when the case is studied at the microscope. When the patient is seen, the laboratory requisition form serves as a source document to record demographic data and notes on the clinical findings. It includes a carbon copy that is sent to the laboratory billing office. The entire report is generated using the computer's word-processing capabilities. Reports longer than one page are rare.

The second report is Swedish. It serves simultaneously as a clinical requisition, a source document, and a form for the final report. It includes several anatomic drawings that the referring physician and the cytopathologist can use to record an illustration of the aspiration site. Hard copies of this document, complete with the drawing, are maintained in the laboratory and in the patient record.

# REFERENCES

1. Borrows GH, Anderson TJ, Lamb JL, Dixon JM: Fine-needle aspiration of breast cancer: Relationship of clinical factors to cytology results in 689 primary malignancies. Cancer 1986;58:1492–1498.
2. Frable WJ: Fine-needle aspiration biopsy: A review. Hum Pathol 1983;14:9–28.
3. Cohen MB, Miller TR, Gonzales JM, Sacks ST, Bottles K: Fine-needle aspiration biopsy: Perceptions of physicians at an academic medical center. Arch Pathol Lab Med 1986;110:813–817.
4. Zajicek J: Aspiration biopsy cytology: II. Cytology of infradiaphragmatic organs. New York: S Karger, 1974.
5. Zajdela A, Ghossein NA, Pilleron JP, et al.: The value of aspiration cytology in the diagnosis of breast cancer: Experience at the Foundation Curie. Cancer 1975;35:499–506.
6. Franzen S, Zajicek J: Aspiration biopsy in the diagnosis of palpable lesions of the breast. Acta Radiol Ther Phys Biol 1968;7:241–262.
7. Hall TL, Layfield LJ, Philippe A, Rosenthal DL: Source of diagnostic error in fine needle aspiration of the thyroid. Cancer 1989;63:718–725.
8. Tao LC, Pierson FG, Delarne NC, Larger B, Sanders DE: Percutaneous fine-needle aspiration biopsy: I. Its value to clinical practice. Cancer 1980;45:1480–1485.
9. Hajdu SI, Melamed MR: Limitations of aspiration cytology in the diagnosis of primary neoplasms. Acta Cytol 1984;28:337–345.
10. Martin HE, Ellis EB: Biopsy by needle puncture and aspiration. Ann Surg 1930;92:169–181.

11. Stewart FW: The diagnosis of tumors by aspiration. Am J Pathol 1933;9:801–815.
12. Soderstrom N: Fine needle aspiration biopsy. New York: Grune & Stratton, 1966.
13. Linsk JA, Franzen S: Fine needle aspiration for the clinician. Philadelphia: Lippincott, 1986.
14. Bell DA, Hajdu SI, Urban JA, Gaston JP: Role of aspiration cytology in the diagnosis and management of mammary lesions in office practice. Cancer 1983;51:1182–1189.
15. VanBogaert L-J, Mazy G: Reliability of the cyto-radioclinical triplet in breast pathology diagnosis. Acta Cytol 1977;21:60–62.
16. Kreuzer G, Boquoi: Aspiration biopsy cytology, mammography and clinical exploration: A modern set up in diagnosis of tumors of the breast. Acta Cytol 1976;20:319–323.
17. Goellner JR, Johnson DA: Cytology of cystic papillary carcinoma of the thyroid. Acta Cytol 1982;26:797–799.
18. Miller JM, Hamburger JI, Taylor CI: Is needle aspiration of the cystic thyroid nodule effective and safe treatment? In: Hamburger, JI, Miller, CI, Eds. Controversies in clinical thyroidology, pp 209–236. New York: Springer-Verlag, 1981.
19. Colacchio TA, LoGerfo P, Feird CR: Fine needle cytologic diagnosis of thyroid nodules: Review and report of 300 cases. Am J Surg 1980;140:568–571.
20. Ramacciotti CE, Pretorius HT, Chu EW, et al.: Diagnostic accuracy and use of aspiration biopsy in the management of thyroid nodules. Arch Intern Med 1984;144:1169–1173.
21. Silverman JF, West RL, Larkin EW, et al.: The role of fine-needle aspiration biopsy in the rapid diagnosis and management of thyroid neoplasms. Cancer 1986;57:1164–1170.
22. VanHerle AJ, Moderator, UCLA conference: The thyroid nodule. Ann Intern Med 1982;96:221–232.
23. Gharib M, Goellner JR, Zinsmeister AR, et al.: Fine needle aspiration biopsy of the thyroid: The problem of suspicious cytologic findings. Ann Intern Med 1984;101:25–28.
24. Esselsyn CB: Aspiration biopsy cytology in diagnosis of thyroid cancer. World J Surg 1981;5:70–71.
25. Hamberger B, Gharib M, Melton LJ, et al.: Fine needle aspiration biopsy of thyroid nodules: Impact on thyroid practice and cost of care. Am J Med 1982;73:381–384.
26. Hawkins F, Bellido D, Bernal C, et al.: Fine needle aspiration biopsy in the diagnosis of thyroid cancer and thyroid disease. Cancer 1987;59:1206–1209.
27. Hutter VP: Goodbye to "fibrocystic disease." N Engl J Med 1985;312:179–181.
28. Dupont WD, Page DL: Risk factors for breast cancer in women with proliferative breast disease. N Engl J Med 1985;312:146–151.
29. Stanley MW: Fine needle aspiration: The ultimate opportunity for the pathologist to act as a clinical consultant. (Syllabus for American Society of Clinical Pathologists Course Number 3404.) Chicago: ASCP Press, 1990.
30. Keen ME, Murad TM, Cohen MI, Matthies JH: Benign breast lesions with malignant clinical and mammographic presentations. Hum Pathol 1985;16:1147–1152.
31. Anderson JA, Gram JB: Radial scar in the female breast: A long-term follow-up study of 32 cases. Cancer 1984;53:2557–2560.
32. Hanna WM, Jambrosic J, Fish E: Aggressive fibromatosis of the breast. Arch Pathol Lab Med 1985;109:260–263.
33. Flint A, Oberman HA: Infarction and squamous metaplasia of intraductal papilloma: A benign breast lesion that may simulate carcinoma. Hum Pathol 1984;15:764–767.
34. Rickert RR, Ralisher L, Hutter RVP: Indurative mastopathy: A benign sclerosing lesion of breast with elastosis which may simulate carcinoma. Cancer 1981;47:561–571.

35. Fenoglio C, Lattes R: Sclerosing papillary proliferations in the female breast: A benign lesion often mistaken for carcinoma. Cancer 1974;33:681–700.

36. Strobel SL, Shah NT, Lucas JG, Tuttle SE: Granular-cell tumor of the breast: A cytologic, immunohistochemical and ultrastructural study of two cases. Acta Cytol 1985;29:598–601.

37. Kline TS, Joshi LP, Neal HS: Fine-needle aspiration of the breast: Diagnosis and pitfalls—A review of 3545 cases. Cancer 1979;44:1458–1464.

38. Strawbridge HTG, Bassett AA, Foldes I: Role of cytology in management of lesions of the breast. Surg Gynecol Obstet 1981;152:1–7.

39. Catania S, Boccato P, Bono A, et al.: Pneumothorax: A rare complication of fine needle aspiration of the breast. Acta Cytol 1989;33:140.

40. Wilson JD, Aiman J, MacDonald PC: The pathogenesis of gynecomastia. Adv Intern Med 1980;25:1–32.

41. Bannayan GA, Hajdu SI: Gynecomastia: Clinicopathologic study of 351 cases. Am J Clin Pathol 1972;57:431–437.

42. Stanley MW, Tani EM, Skoog L: Mucinous breast carcinoma and mixed mucinous/infiltrating ductal carcinoma: A comparative cytologic study. Diagn Cytopathol 1989;5:134–138.

43. Wargotz ES, Silverberg SG: Medullary carcinoma of the breast: A clinicopathologic study with appraisal of current diagnostic criteria. Hum Pathol 1988;19:1340–1346.

44. Stanley MW, Tani EM, Skoog L: Fine needle aspiration of fibroadenomas of the breast with atypia: A spectrum including cases which cytologically mimic carcinoma. Diagn Cytopathol 1990;6:375–382.

45. Layfield LJ, Glasgow DJ, DuPuis MH: Fine-needle aspiration of lymphadenopathy of suspected infectious etiology. Arch Pathol Lab Med 1985;109:810–812.

46. Robert FJ, Linsey S: The value of microbial cultures in diagnostic lymph node biopsy. J Infect Dis 1984;149:162–165.

47. Bottles K, McPhaul LW, Volbesding P: Fine-needle aspiration biopsy of patients with the acquired immunodeficiency syndrome (AIDS): Experience in an outpatient clinic. Ann Intern Med 1988;108:42–45.

48. Stanley MW, Burton LG, Horwitz CA: Atypical mycobacterial infection in fine needle aspiration smears from lymph nodes in patients with the acquired immunodeficiency syndrome: A distinctive cytologic appearance. Diagn Cytopathol 1990;6:118–121.

49. Kline TS, Rannan V, Kline IR: Lymphadenopathy and aspiration biopsy cytology: Review of 376 superficial nodes. Cancer 1984;54:1076–1081.

50. Engzell U, Jakobsson PA, Sigurdson A, Zajicek J. Aspiration biopsy of metastatic carcinoma in lymph nodes of the neck: A review of 1101 consecutive cases. Acta Otolaryngol 1971;72:138–147.

51. Betsill WL, Hajdu SI: Percutaneous aspiration biopsy of lymph nodes. Am J Clin Pathol 1980;73:471–479.

52. Kline TS, Rannan V: Aspiration biopsy cytology and melanoma. Am J Clin Pathol 1982;77:597–601.

53. Friedman M, Forgione H, Shanbhag V: Needle aspiration of metastatic melanoma. Acta Cytol 1980;24:7–15.

54. Woyke S, Domagala W, Czerniak B, Strokowsky M: Fine needle aspiration cytology of malignant melanoma of the skin. Acta Cytol 1980;24:529–538.

55. Lee RE, Valaitis J, Ralis O., et al.: Lymph node examination by fine needle aspiration in patients with known or suspected malignancy. Acta Cytol 1987;31:563–72.

56. Robb-Smith AHT, Taylor CR: Lymph node biopsy, p. 10. New York: Oxford University Press, 1981.

57. Hajdu SI, Melamed MR: The diagnostic value of aspiration smears. Am J Clin Pathol 1973;59:350–356.

58. Tani EM, Christensson B, Pornit A, Skoog L: Immunocytochemical analysis and cytomorphologic diagnosis on fine needle aspirates of lymphoproliferative disease. Acta Cytol 1988;32:209–215.

59. Skoog L, Tani E: The role of fine-needle aspiration cytology in the diagnosis of non-Hodgkin's lymphoma. Diagn Oncol 1991;1:12–18.

60. Stanley MW, Steeper TA, Horwitz CA, et al.: Fine-needle aspiration of lymph nodes in patients with acute infectious mononucleosis. Diagn Cytopathol 1990;6:323–329.

61. Linsk JA, Franzen S: Clinical aspiration cytology. 2nd ed, p. 351. Cambridge, England: Lippincott, 1989.

62. Friedman M, Kim CL, Shimaoka K, et al.: Appraisal of aspiration cytology in management of Hodgkin's disease. Cancer 1980;45:1653–1667.

63. Pontiflex AH, Klimo P: Application of aspiration biopsy cytology to lymphomas. Cancer 1984;53:553–556.

64. Mavec P, Eneroth CM, Franzen S, et al.: Aspiration biopsy of salivary gland tumors: I. Correlation of cytologic reports from 652 aspirations with clinical and histologic findings. Acta Otolaryngol 1964;58:472–484.

65. O'Dwyer P, Farrar WB, James AG, et al.: Needle aspiration biopsy of major salivary gland tumors. Cancer 1986;57:554–557.

66. Engzell U, Esposti PL, Rubio C, et al.: Investigation of tumor spread in connection with aspiration biopsy. Acta Radiol 1971;10:385–398.

67. Eneroth CM, Zajicek J: Aspiration biopsy of salivary gland tumors: III. Morphologic studies on smears and histologic sections from 360 mixed tumors. Acta Cytol 1966;10:440–454.

68. Cohen MB, Ljung B-ME, Boles R: Salivary gland tumors: Fine-needle aspiration vs. frozen-section diagnosis. Acta Otolaryngol 1986;112:867–869.

69. Qizilbash AH, Young JEM: Guides to clinical aspiration biopsy: Head and neck. New York: Igaku-Shoin Medical, 1968. pp. 15–19.

70. Kovacic J, Rainer S, Levicnik A: Aspiration cytology of normal structures and non-neoplastic cysts of the ovary. In: Blaustein A, ed. Pathology of the female genital tract. 2nd ed., pp. 716–724. New York: Springer-Verlag, 1982.

71. Kovacic J, Raines S, Levicnik A, Cizelj T: Cytology of benign ovarian lesions in connection with laparoscopy. In: Zajicek J, ed. Aspiration biopsy cytology: Part 2. Cytology of intradiaphragmatic organs, pp. 58–61. Basel, Switzerland: Karger, 1979.

72. Kjellgren O, Angstrom T, Bergman F, Wiklund D-E: Fine needle aspiration biopsy in diagnosis and classification of ovarian carcinoma. Cancer 1971;28:967–976.

73. Geier GR, Strecker JR: Aspiration cytology and E2 content in ovarian tumors. Acta Cytol 1981;25:400–406.

74. Ganjei P, Nadji M: Aspiration cytology of ovarian neoplasms: A review. Acta Cytol 1984;28:329–332.

75. Diernaes E, Rasmussen J, Sorensen T, Hasch E: Ovarian cyts: Management by puncture? Lancet 1987;2:1084.

76. Christopherson WM: Cytologic detection and diagnosis of cancer: Its contributions and limitations. Cancer 1983;51:1201-1208.

77. Koss LG, Woyke S, Olszewski W: Aspiration biopsy: Cytologic interpretation and histologic bases. p. 416. New York: Igaku-Shoin, 1984.

78. Esposti PL, Elman A, Norlen H: Complications of transrectal aspiration of the prostate. Scand J Urol Nephrol 1975;9:208–212.

79. Chodak GW, Seinberg GD, Bibbo M, et al.: The role of transrectal aspiration in the diagnosis of prostatic cancer. J Urol 1986;135:299–302.

80. Stanley MW, Hedlund PO, Ronstrom L, et al.: Determination of false negative rate in fine-needle aspiration of prostate: Study of sequential aspirations in 30 untreated carcinoma patients. Urol 1989;34:73–75.

81. Kaye KW, Horwitz CA: Transrectal fine needle biopsy of the prostate: Combined histological and cytological technique. J Urol 1988;139:1229–1231.

82. Kaye KW, Horwitz CA: Transrectal ultrasound-guided prostate biopsies using new automatic gun: Analysis of 100 consecutive cases. J Endourol 1989;3:155–161.

83. Kline TJ, Kline TS: Communication and cytopathology: Part II. Malpractice. Diagn Cytopathol 1991;7:227–228.

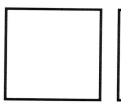

# Clinical Examples of
# Fine-Needle Aspiration

**3**

## THE NATURE OF CYTOLOGIC DIAGNOSES IN FINE-NEEDLE ASPIRATION

Cytologic diagnoses generally fall into one of two categories: (1) complete, specific diagnoses, and (2) less-specific diagnoses of benign versus malignant masses. The first is complete classification of the disease process, which yields the same type of diagnosis rendered by study of histologic material. This is commonly achieved in a variety of settings for which a neoplasm, infection, or inflammatory process can be defined as fully by FNA as would be possible with any other morphologic preparation requiring human interpretation of visual information.

Examples include fibroadenoma of the breast, adenocarcinoma of the prostate, benign mixed tumors of the parotid, and lymph-node hyperplasia. In other instances, a complete evaluation occurs when initial cytologic findings are extended by ICC, lymphocyte surface-marker analysis, or culture of microorganisms. This type of diagnosis is especially useful when applied during the primary-care phase of a patient's workup. Specific benign diagnoses lead to medical treatment, limited surgical procedures, or observation of the lesion over time. A malignant diagnosis results in referral to the most appropriate specialist and to highly selected application of other diagnostic or staging modalities.

The second type of diagnosis that can come from FNA is less specific, but may answer immediately the fundamental question of whether the mass is benign or malignant. This increases follow-up options for many masses found in the thyroid, lymph nodes, breast, and other sites. It is especially helpful in evaluation of lesions noted in patients with a prior history of malignancy. The alternatives to recurrent malignancy generally include reactive or infectious lesions that may arise de novo or as a result of therapy (surgery, radiation, etc.).

This less specific type of diagnosis may give a list of differential diagnostic possibilities. A lymph-node aspiration may yield malignant cells that, although impossible to characterize fully, can be recognized as neoplastic, malignant, not lymphoma, metastatic, and possibly originating in one of two or three designated body sites. A thyroid specimen may represent the very small group of cases in which it is not possible to distinguish a follicular adenoma from a follicular carcinoma. For the uncommon individual with this problem, surgery is required, but when FNA is applied as a primary-care device to the large number of thyroid enlargements in the general population, many will be excluded from surgery. Furthermore, for this patient, a very simple, rapid, safe, and painless FNA will have accomplished great diagnostic leaps by having ruled out various possibilities, indicating that the abnormal gland is *not* any of the following: colloid goiter, thyroiditis, papillary carcinoma, a lymph node mistaken for thyroid disease, or a rare malignancy such as thyroid lymphoma, medullary carcinoma, or metastatic carcinoma.

This second type of diagnosis, while less complete than the first, is nevertheless of immense clinical utility. This is most true when FNA is applied early in the patient's evaluation and is considered as a primary-care device applicable to virtually all palpable masses. This approach allows great benefits in cost, time, and decreased suffering to accrue to the patient. As was just illustrated, the results may come in the form of exclusions, recommendations, and greatly reduced numbers of possible diseases for the physician to investigate.

Such basic distinctions as lymphoma versus carcinoma are readily accomplished by FNA. In some instances, these results will not yield ultimate, detailed subclassification of the tumor; that must be left to the histopathologists. This does not detract from the fact that (1) the patient will have been immediately sent to the best type of specialized care; (2) costly, time-consuming, and possibly painful procedures may be avoided; (3) delay in diagnosis (and its medicolegal consequences) by following lesions that turn out to be malignant will not occur; and (4) the histopathologists receive warning about special studies that may be needed for final tumor classification.

Thus, from a clinical—especially a primary care—perspective, it is not necessary that FNA be required to yield histopathology-like perfection in tumor diagnosis and classification. For the clinician, FNA will often function as a triage device. For the pathologist, it may be somewhat like a rapid-frozen section. (The utility of the latter analogy is borne out by the recent expansion of interest and research in the use of intraoperative cytology, both by FNA and by imprints of surgical specimens.)

Those who study FNA and then demean the method by focusing on its limitations in tumor classification fail to realize that it was created to be a primary care, first-line technique. Their writings usually point out difficulty in cytologic classification of uncommon lesions. This does have some value and underscores the need for circumspection in diagnostic cytopathology. On the other hand, the majority of patients to whom FNA is applicable suffer from relatively common problems that are readily recognized or triaged by cytologic means.

# COMMENTS ON SPECIMEN ADEQUACY

Chapter 1 and the upcoming case studies illustrate the generous material that is often obtained by FNA. Methods for preparing high-quality smears from abundant specimens were discussed in Chapter 2. In such instances, it is not necessary to consider whether an aspiration has given sufficient material for meaningful diagnosis.

Some cases, however, raise the issue of specimen adequacy. Benign fibrocystic breast lesions often yield scant material. Aspirations from endocrine organs (thyroid) may dilute any cellular material in blood. Cyst fluids may be extremely hypocellular. Colloid goiter of the thyroid may yield grossly obvious colloid that contains very few cells when studied at the microscope. Aspiration of some carcinomas may show mostly necrosis, with very few viable cells. In the proper clinical setting, each of these and other types of cell-poor specimens may be not only adequate for interpretation, but also highly diagnostic.

Detailed analysis of specimen adequacy for any body site is beyond the scope of this book. In general, however, decisions about adequacy must include reflections on several factors, including (1) the site of the aspiration, (2) the clinical findings, (3) possible radiographic features, (4) observations made at the time of aspiration as the lesion is punctured by the needle, (5) the nature of material expressed onto the slide before smearing, and (6) the overall quality of the FNA procedure, as reflected in the experience of the operator. Only then does microscope evaluation of adequacy have meaning relevant to the patient's condition.

Knowing that the mass has been securely stabilized and that accurate needle placement has been achieved contributes greatly to the assessment of specimen adequacy. Correlation of clinical findings with the gross appearance and quantity of material recovered and with any change in texture as the mass is punctured by the needle further enhances the knowledge that the most adequate possible specimen has been obtained.

Thus, determinations of specimen adequacy and the completeness of the FNA process depend heavily on observations made at the bedside. Efforts to express specimen adequacy solely in terms of the number of punctures performed, the number of smears prepared or the number of cell groups observed seem to us misguided and simplistic. The cases discussed in this chapter provide examples of these principles.

If expert, careful technique has been used to ensure accurate puncture and thorough sampling of the palpable abnormality, and if well-prepared material has been carefully examined, then optimum application of FNA will have occurred. Clinical and radiographic considerations may then lead to further investigation.

# CASE STUDIES IN FINE-NEEDLE ASPIRATION

The methods and concepts developed in Chapters 1 and 2 are now illustrated with 10 case studies. All are drawn from the practice of one of the authors (MWS). All were aspirated with 25-gauge needles, and in each case, results were available to the referring clinician within 30 minutes of our being called to see the patient.

The cases have been selected to emphasize technical and clinical aspects of FNA, including assessment prior to puncture, radiographic evaluation, consultation with other physicians, and use of microbiologic evaluation where appropriate. The diagnostic considerations include identification of malignancies and their therapeutically significant subclassification. Two studies illustrate staging of advanced carcinomas by aspiration of metastatic deposits. Diagnosis of benign lesions where metastases had been expected is also illustrated.

This brief essay describes only a small number of many successful FNA applications. We hope to suggest the wide range of clinical problems to which the method can be applied.

As much as we have stressed that FNA is a useful primary means of diagnosing palpable masses, one of our themes throughout this book has been that, like any other medical test, it has limitations. Our goal has been to minimize errors by optimizing technique. We have emphasized that good clinical judgment is the ultimate barrier against the consequences of incomplete or inaccurate diagnoses. It is fitting that Case 10 closes this treatise with histopathologically defined reasons for FNA's failure to recognize various examples of lymph-node pathology.

Wider application of FNA will benefit many patients and will conserve resources only if it is technically optimized and practiced in the light of prudent clinical judgment.

## Case 1

### Clinical History

A 58-year-old woman was referred for needle aspiration of a 2 cm, readily palpable breast mass. The patient discovered this mass herself but delayed seeking medical attention for 3 months. Her gynecologist referred her to an experienced surgeon, who felt that the lesion was probably malignant, based on physical examination. She was otherwise in good health. Neither axillary nor supraclavicular lymphadenopathy was detected.

The patient arrived at the FNA clinic bringing a brief note from the referring physician. This contained a description of the physical findings, including the location of the lesion. The cytopathologist's examination confirmed these findings, which were also considered suggestive of breast carcinoma.

### Fine-Needle Aspiration

This was a very straightforward problem in both clinical and technical terms. The mass was easily localized and stabilized. Two aspirations were performed with 25-gauge (0.5 mm) needles. Each yielded sufficient material for preparing three smears; both dried and spray-fixed slides were thus available.

The same firm, desmoplastic tumor stroma that gave the mass its characteristic presentation at physical examination enabled the operator to feel the needle's entry into the neoplasm. This was an important step in ensuring accurate sampling.

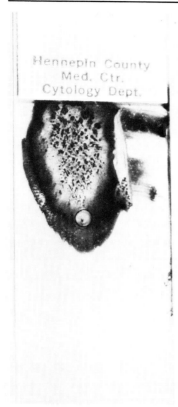

Figure 3.1.
*This stained smear from aspiration of a breast carcinoma shows numerous large tissue particles.*

Once material had been obtained and spread onto glass slides, it was grossly inspected. As is often the case in this clinical setting, numerous grossly visible tissue particles were recovered. When uncontaminated by large amounts of blood, these appear white or gray. Recovery of this type of material is very unusual in benign breast lesions. It may be seen in fibroadenoma, but in such cases, the physical and microscopic findings will usually differ from those of carcinoma. Identification of abundant tissue was further evidence that accurate puncture and thorough sampling had been achieved. The stained smear also showed numerous tissue particles (Figure 3.1).

By attending to the texture of tissues passed by the needle and by inspecting the aspirated material, it was possible to leave the bedside knowing that a diagnostic specimen had been obtained. The problem depicted in Figure 1.2 was avoided. Special studies are not commonly required, so that repeat aspirations are rare in this setting.

### Cytologic Findings

All smears were highly cellular and featured malignant cells, both singly and in groups (Figure 3.2 and 3.3). A secure diagnosis of carcinoma was rendered.[1]

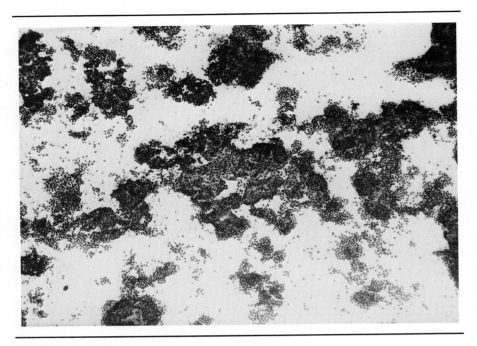

Figure 3.2.
*This microscopic view of the smear depicted in Figure 3.1 shows large tissue particles. Between them are single cells that have been spread thinly and are suitable for detailed microscopic study (Papanicolaou Stain, ×50 before a 34% reduction). Very little blood is present.*

### Clinical Impact of FNA

With a firm tissue diagnosis in hand, the surgeon was able to help the patient begin to deal with any problems of denial that she may have had. When physician and patient agreed that a malignancy was present, possible therapeutic options and prognostic implications were addressed fully. The patient made an informed decision regarding the several treatments available today. Optimum counseling took place before any surgery was performed. Most two-stage operations in which separate procedures are used for diagnosis and for definitive therapy can be avoided by preoperative cytologic diagnosis.

Authorities differ as to whether cytologic diagnoses of breast carcinoma should be confirmed by frozen section at the time of surgery. Some view this as a redundancy that wastes resources, while others consider it to be a useful quality-assurance device. Silverman et al. have provided a careful assessment of this subject, including a detailed cost analysis.[2] Decisions about this complex issue must ultimately be made by surgeons and pathologists. We agree with Frable that frozen-section confirmation should not be viewed as an affront to the cytopathologist's skill.[3] Our common goal is the best possible care of our patients.

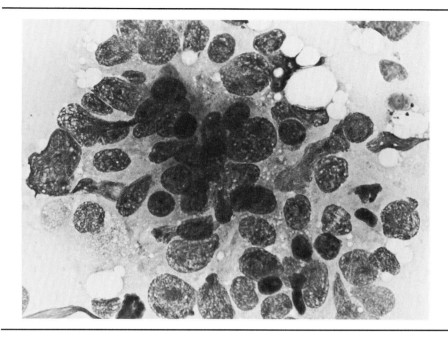

Figure 3.3.
*At higher magnification, this smear shows numerous loosely clustered tumor cells. Each has an intact rim of cytoplasm (modified Diff-Quik® stain, X788 before a 34% reduction).*

## Case 2

### Clinical History

This 60-year-old woman had mild diffuse lumpiness of both breasts, without dominant masses. Routine mammography disclosed an area of approximately 8 mm diameter with changes strongly suggestive of carcinoma. She was referred to a surgical oncologist with extensive experience and interest in breast malignancy. By directing the physical examination to the area identified by the mammographer, a small area of firmness was detected.

The guidelines for applying FNA (see Table 2.2) make it clear that one should not attempt aspiration of mammographic findings that are not associated with a palpable mass. (Stereotactic, radiographically directed aspiration of such lesions is now possible, using a special apparatus, but this complex subject is not considered further here.)

In this case, however, careful consultation among team members, including the mammographer, the surgeon, and the cytopathologist allowed directed aspiration of a subtle physical finding. The radiographs permitted selection of one from among several seemingly minor breast abnormalities. Both the physical

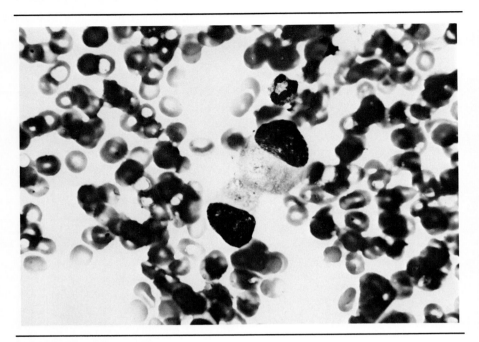

Figure 3.4.
*Cytologic smears from this very small breast mass show scattered malignant cells. These have a signet-ring appearance with eccentric nuclei and a single cytoplasmic vacuole (modified Diff-Quik® stain, ×788 before a 34% reduction).*

examination and the FNA (described next) were facilitated by the soft (fatty) rather than firm (fibrous) nature of the background breast tissue.

### Fine-Needle Aspiration

The procedure was carefully executed, following all of the steps outlined in Table 2.3. Radiologist, surgeon, and cytopathologist first discussed the case at the x-ray viewbox. Examination of the radiographically indicated area was then carried out. The physical findings were not indicative of malignancy, but the subtle palpable abnormality was agreed on.

FNA was carried out with a 25-gauge (0.5 mm) needle of 1.5 inches (3.8 cm) length. Probing a cone-shaped volume of tissue (see Figure 1.14) showed that most of the local breast tissue was soft (fatty). An area of firmness was located by careful repeated probing with the needle, and aspiration was directed at this finding. The return was bloody, without grossly visible tissue particles. Smears were prepared and dried. A rapid Romanowsky stain (modified Diff-Quik® staining; Table 1.6) was applied and examined immediately, using a temporary coverslip mounted with water, as described in Chapter 1.

### Cytologic Findings

Tumor cells were scattered over the smear in a background of red blood cells. They were seen singly and in couplets (Figure 3.4). They featured large, irregularly shaped, eccentrically located nuclei and abundant cytoplasm. A cytoplasmic vacuole suggestive of lumen formation or secretory activity was frequently present. A diagnosis of carcinoma was made.

### Clinical Impact of FNA

The patient elected local excision and postoperative radiation therapy. The mass was excised completely, with a surrounding margin of uninvolved tissue. Figure 3.5 shows a whole-mount section demonstrating the very small size (8 mm) and fibrotic nature of this carcinoma. The fibrosis probably accounts for the low cellularity of the aspirate. Histologic sections showed infiltrating, usually single malignant cells with the same signet-ring morphology seen in the smear material (Figure 3.6).

This case illustrates a rather extreme example of aspirating a minimally palpable lesion. Successful results depended on close consultation among members of a team of three physicians from different specialties. This multidisciplinary approach to identification, evaluation, and treatment of breast lesions has been successfully used in many institutions.

This case also highlights other issues of clinical management of patients with abnormal findings in the breast. All three methods of evaluation were skillfully applied (physical examination, mammography, and FNA). The radiographic and cytologic findings provided compelling evidence of malignancy. Patient counseling and treatment were instituted with minimal delay.

Figure 3.5.
*Whole-mount sections show a small (0.8 mm) breast carcinoma surrounded by fatty tissue (hematoxylin and eosin [H&E]; whole mount).*

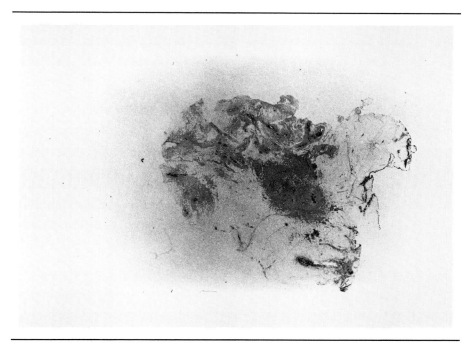

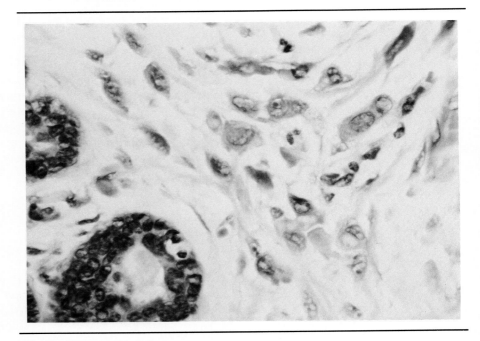

Figure 3.6.
*Tissue sections from this small breast carcinoma show infiltration by single malignant cells. These have morphology similar to that illustrated cytologically in Figure 3.4. Normal ducts can be seen at the lower left (H&E, ×500 before a 34% reduction).*

If the FNA had been nondiagnostic, the patient would have fit into the third category in Table 2–7. Diagnostic surgical biopsy would have been needed. The usual way to accomplish this would have been with a wire localization. In this procedure, the radiologist places a wire in or near the lesion, using mammographic guidance. This wire then guides the surgeon to the lesion. FNA provided an alternative method of diagnosis at considerable savings in time, cost, and patient discomfort.

## Case 3

### Clinical History

Our third case also represents a breast mass. This 68-year-old woman was referred for evaluation of a 6-cm tumor. Both the referring surgeon and the cytopathologist felt that the physical findings were entirely consistent with carcinoma. No axillary adenopathy was detected. The patient was otherwise in good health.

### Fine-Needle Aspiration

The technical aspects of localization, stabilization, aspiration, and specimen preparation were in no way out of the ordinary. Abundant tissue was obtained.

*Cytologic Findings*

Both epithelial and stromal elements were present. The former consisted of flat sheets with uniform ductal cells arranged in the honeycomb pattern that typifies the cytology of many benign glandular epithelia (Figure 3.7). The stromal tissue was very different from the hypocellular collagenous fragments often seen in FNA specimens from fibroadenomas or areas of nonneoplastic fibrous tissue. These tissue fragments showed a highly cellular spindle cell proliferation (Figure 3.8). A diagnosis of phyllodes tumor was rendered.

*Clinical Impact of FNA*

If reasonable technical standards are observed, one is virtually certain of obtaining tissue from a mass such as this. The cytology was clearly not that of carcinoma. The finding of benign epithelium and cellular stroma is the expected picture in phyllodes tumor. (Use of the sometimes misleading term *cystosarcoma* is to be discouraged. Furthermore, the complex distinction between benign and malignant phyllodes tumors is beyond the scope of our current interests.)

In this patient, with what was by clinical criteria a typical case of breast carcinoma, an alternative diagnosis was made preoperatively by FNA. While most masses that appear to represent breast carcinoma are ultimately typical of this entity, surprises do occur. Granular cell tumor, fat necrosis, and other benign masses may clinically and radiographically mimic carcinoma very strongly. Making a preoperative diagnosis often alters the surgical approach considerably.

Figure 3.7.
*Benign duct cells in a honeycomb arrangement form a flat sheet (modified Diff-Quik®
stain, ×500 before a 34% reduction).*

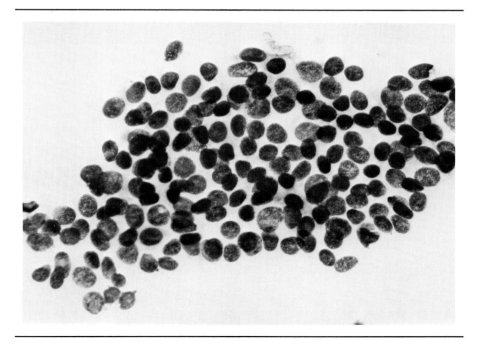

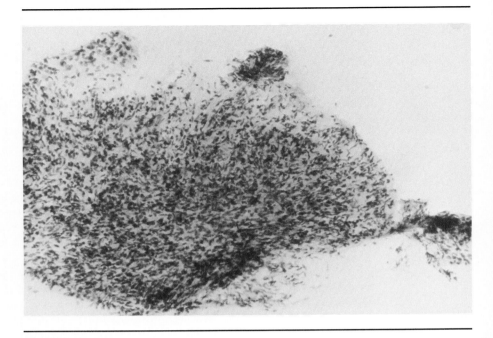

Figure 3.8.
*Cellular stromal fragments (Papanicolaou stain, X125 before a 28% reduction).*

The purpose of this case presentation is not to discuss the highly variable cytopathology of phyllodes tumor.[4] However, simply showing the mass to represent anything other than typical breast carcinoma will suffice to initiate further clinical evaluation, including surgical biopsy or frozen-section evaluation prior to definitive excision.

The natural history of phyllodes tumors includes local recurrence. Only 10 percent of cases metastasize to the lungs, bones, or the central nervous system. Thus, the surgical approach differs from that usually applied to breast carcinoma because axillary lymph-node sampling is usually unnecessary.

Unexpected diagnoses occur in other body sites as well. In Chapter 2, we discussed the comments of Qizilbash and Young regarding salivary-gland FNA. These authors found that surprises tended to occur in those cases that seemed least problematic at initial clinical evaluation. Preoperative evaluation by FNA can improve the clinical approach to lesions that provide such a surprise. A significant improvement in clinical decision making can occur, even without a final specific cytologic diagnosis.

## Case 4

### Clinical History

This 64-year-old female had undergone a modified radical mastectomy for infiltrating ductal carcinoma 2 years earlier. Her incision scar was well healed and showed no associated masses. Several centimeters above the scar was a single, firm, dermal nodule. This 3 mm × 5 mm lesion was slightly pale but was more easily located by palpation than by inspection. It was most apparent when the fingers were passed lightly over the patient's skin.

This type of lesion was described in Chapter 2 and is strongly suggestive of a dermal recurrence of breast carcinoma. These small nodules resemble rice grains.

### Fine-Needle Aspiration

In Chapter 2, technical problems in aspirating small dermal nodules were described. The technique illustrated in Figures 2.24 and 2.25 was applied. A small droplet of thick white material was obtained. This was split so that both a dry slide and a spray-fixed slide could be prepared. The characteristic rotten-egg odor of the keratinous cyst was noted.

### Cytologic Findings

Both smears showed large numbers of mature, anucleate squamous cells (Figure 3.9). No inflammation, microorganisms, or malignant cells were present. The bedside impression of keratinous cyst was confirmed. The patient remains without evidence of recurrence 1 year later.

Figure 3.9.
*Smears from this keratinous cyst show large numbers of mature, anucleate squamous cells. Their sharp cell borders and translucent cytoplasm give such cell groups a mosaic pattern (Papanicolaou stain, ×400 before a 34% reduction).*

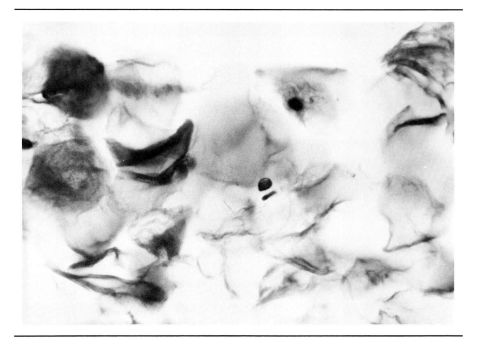

### Clinical Impact of FNA

Dermal recurrence of breast carcinoma is an ominous prognostic sign. Excision under local anesthesia would have given the same diagnostic results, but FNA provided the information at a cost much lower than would be possible with local excision, tissue processing, and histologic evaluation. Results were available in minutes rather than overnight (or over the weekend). Both patients and physicians appreciate such rapid resolution of a very frightening clinical problem.

## Case 5

### Clinical History

A 70-year-old male was noted to have a solitary 3-cm, peripheral, left-lung mass on chest radiograph. Clinical options for follow-up ranged from doing nothing (as might be prudent in an older individual with medical problems) to surgical excision. The latter option would be appropriate in a healthy patient with no evidence of metastatic disease in whom a curative resection might be possible.

Evaluation for possible metastatic deposits could include physical examination and various radiographic studies. In this case, a left supraclavicular mass was palpable. This 1.5 cm lesion was firm, rounded, and mobile. It was thus compatible with an enlarged lymph node and was chosen as a target for FNA. If the tissue obtained had not provided a reasonable diagnosis for the lung mass, a radiographic search for metastases and FNA of the lung mass would have been considered.

### Fine-Needle Aspiration

Technically, this represented a straightforward study of a palpably enlarged lymph node. As noted in Chapter 2, aspiration of the supraclavicular area carries a small risk of pneumothorax because the lung reaches above the level of the clavicle. The lymph nodes lie in tissue planes superficial to the pulmonary cupola. Careful attention to the changes in tissue texture as the needle enters the lesion will help prevent advancing too far.

The aspirated material was grossly consistent with the yield one expects from a metastatic carcinoma. Minimally bloody, glistening gray tissue particles were recovered. When smears were prepared, these particles dispersed easily, in a manner consistent with poorly cohesive tissue fragments. This is often seen with malignant neoplasms (such as the metastatic carcinoma suspected in this case) or with lymphoid tissue.

This observation can help distinguish a useful puncture from one that has yielded particles of skeletal muscle. The latter is sometimes obtained during technically difficult aspirations, especially in the neck. The first clue that one has missed the lesion comes when the aspiration is painful for the patient. Most lymph node or thyroid punctures produce a brief sharp pain as the skin is pierced. Aspiration of the target lesion is usually not painful.

Aspiration of muscle may yield grossly impressive tissue particles. Unlike those described previously, however, these are very resilient. Rather than being dispersed as the smears are prepared, they immediately recoil to their round or cylindrical shape as they pop out from behind the advancing edge of the spreader slide. They are usually present in a background of blood that lacks the granular, cloudy, or necrotic appearance commonly recognized when malignancies are spread out on a slide.

This type of careful attention to detail as the smears are prepared helps one recognize and repeat immediately some inadequate aspirations. This is one of the reasons outlined in Table 2.1 for suggesting that a single individual perform the procedure and evaluate the cytology. Such individuals have the combined clinical and microscopic experience to become skilled in this type of assessment.

### Cytologic Findings

The cells illustrated in Figure 2.18 are representative of this case. Cell groups and single cells showed moderate amounts of cytoplasm, prominent nucleoli, distinct nuclear chromatin, and irregularities of nuclear shape. The irregularities included both notchlike indentations and lobulations. These were typical of adenocarcinoma and were compatible with origin in the lung.[5]

### Clinical Impact of FNA

The diagnosis of metastatic adenocarcinoma in a supraclavicular lymph node adequately explained the physical and radiographic findings in this patient. Furthermore, the staging information provided by identifying this malignancy in a nodal metastasis clearly eliminated any consideration of surgically curing the lung mass. If clinically needed, additional staging information could be obtained by radiographic means without resorting to costly, painful surgical procedures that would not improve the patient's ultimate outcome.

This type of simultaneous diagnosis and staging is a common application of FNA. It represents a rapid and extremely humane way to obtain this information in patients for whom little or no effective treatment may be available.

Other means of evaluating this patient would have included surgical excision of the supraclavicular node, FNA of the lung mass with radiographic guidance, and thoracotomy with excision of the mass. The low cost and rapidity of bedside FNA, as well as the extremely low complication rate for this procedure, clearly make it the method of choice for this type of patient.

## Case 6

### Clinical History

This 65-year-old male, with a history of cigarette smoking, was found to have a large lung mass associated with enlargement of mediastinal lymph nodes (Figure 3.10). CT scan also showed multiple liver masses consistent with metastatic carcinoma (Figure 3.11). The liver was palpably enlarged and extended 4 cm below the inferior costal margin in the right upper quadrant.

Although several possible infectious or neoplastic diagnoses could have been suggested for this patient, it was highly probable that he suffered from small cell anaplastic (oat cell) carcinoma of the lung, with metastases in mediastinal lymph nodes and the liver. Confirmation of this diagnosis by the simplest possible means is always in order because its treatment is based on chemical therapy or radiotherapy without surgical intervention.

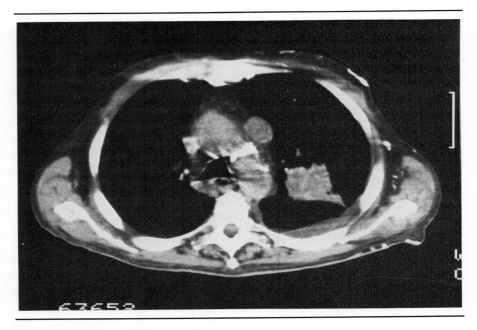

Figure 3.10.
*This CT scan shows a large lung mass associated with mediastinal adenopathy. (Photograph courtesy of Dr. John Knoedler, Hennepin County Medical Center, Minneapolis, Minnesota)*

Obtaining tissue from the lung would have provided a diagnosis. Sampling of the liver would yield both diagnostic and staging information. Possible approaches included bronchoscopy, thoracotomy, mediastinoscopy, core liver biopsy, laparoscopic liver biopsy or aspiration, lung aspiration, or percutaneous liver aspiration. Percutaneous liver FNA would be the least costly and the most rapid. If diagnostic tissue were not obtained, one of the other methods could then have been used. FNA would not have introduced significant delay or expenditures.

### Fine-Needle Aspiration

With the abdominal CT scans available for review, it was determined that pathological hepatic tissue lay immediately deep to the abdominal wall in the right upper quadrant. No intervening lung tissue was present in this area. The enlarged liver was easily located below the inferior costal margin by palpation and percussion.

In elderly patients with a history of smoking, the danger of pneumothorax must be considered. It is these individuals whose compromised lung function gives this rare complication of FNA its greatest danger. Careful study of the CT scan can assure the physician that the site chosen for puncture is not overlaid by pulmonary tissue.

In patients with diffuse hepatic involvement by metastatic disease, it is often unnecessary to use radiographic guidance during FNA. Review of tomographic anatomy and pathology as just outlined makes it safe and reasonable to aspirate

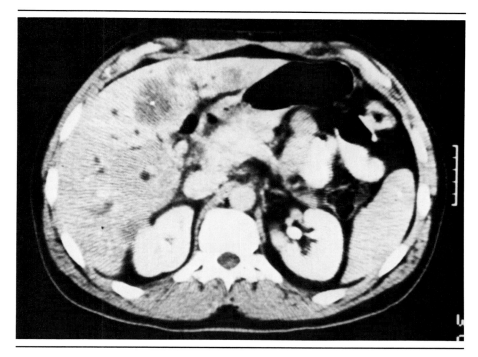

Figure 3.11.
*This abdominal CT scan shows extensive involvement of the liver by nodules consistent with metastatic carcinoma. (Photograph courtesy of Dr. John Knoedler, Hennepin County Medical Center, Minneapolis, Minnesota)*

the enlarged liver at the bedside. We use a 25-gauge (0.5 mm) needle with either 2-inch (5 cm) or 3½-inch (8.8 cm) length. Prior to this procedure, coagulation studies should be obtained. In the event of significant hemorrhage, it may not be possible adequately to apply pressure to the aspiration site (see following discussion).

The FNA technique borrows technical points from the method for biopsy of the liver with larger cutting needles. The area of intended aspiration is located, and the skin is prepared with alcohol. (The labeled slides, syringe pistol, syringe, needles, and slide fixatives are already at the bedside.)

The patient is asked to breathe slowly and not too deeply. After several breaths, the patient is asked to stop breathing for a few seconds, during which the puncture is performed. It is important that the patient be told to "just stop breathing" and not to take in a deep breath. We describe this breathing method before the aspiration is executed. Some patients may need to practice briefly to achieve good results. When the needle is withdrawn, the patient is instructed to breathe normally, and pressure is applied to the puncture site as smears are prepared.

This method of breathing stops the normal respiratory excursions of the liver during the aspiration. It also minimizes the volume of potentially intrusive lung tissue. Thus, safety, accuracy, and technical ease are achieved by these simple means.

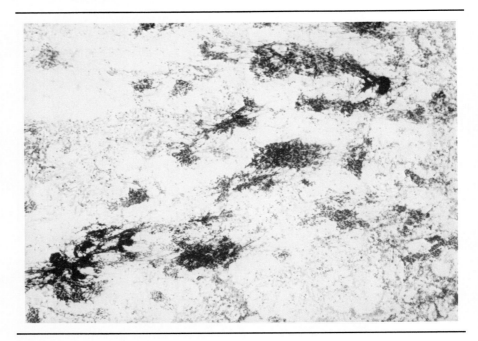

Figure 3.12.
*At low magnification, numerous tissue particles are seen in this liver aspiration (Papanicolaou stain, ×50 before a 34% reduction).*

The patient described previously was approached by this method. A single puncture yielded material sufficient to prepare four smears. Two were spray-fixed, and two were air-dried.

### Cytologic Findings

All smears were highly cellular, with a background of necrotic cells. While nonspecific, necrosis is an expected feature of small-cell anaplastic carcinoma. Large tissue fragments were also present (Figure 3.12). Closer examination showed small cells in cohesive tissue fragments. Individual cells showed scant cytoplasm, molding to adjacent cells, nuclear hyperchromasia (dark staining), and coarse chromatin granules (Figure 3.13). These features were diagnostic of small-cell anaplastic carcinoma. Large amounts of tissue were available for study, but even in low numbers, these cell groups are highly characteristic of this neoplasm.[6]

### Clinical Impact of FNA

This case is similar to Case 5, in that both illustrate simultaneous diagnosis and staging of a malignancy by bedside FNA. This case is somewhat more complex, in that liver aspiration without radiographic guidance was employed. Using the safeguards just discussed, this was a procedure of very low risk. We have used it to diagnose metastases of carcinoma and malignant melanoma, as well as

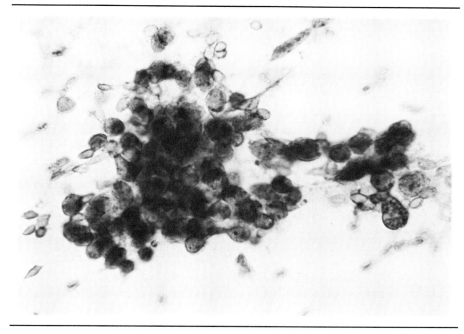

Figure 3.13.
*This liver aspiration shows small-cell anaplastic (oat cell) carcinoma with darkly staining nuclei and scant cytoplasm. The tumor cells form a cohesive tissue fragment (Papanicolaou stain, ×500 before a 34% reduction).*

disseminated histoplasmosis. Currently, FNA has no role to play in the evaluation of metabolic liver disease, although it has been suggested that hepatic iron overload can be studied in FNA material.[7]

We have seen patients with this neoplasm present with the same findings as this individual, plus superior vena cava syndrome. Diagnosis by FNA allows emergency therapy to be initiated immediately after admission.

Following this type of percutaneous liver aspiration, the patient should be observed for several hours. If not hospitalized, he or she should be kept in the clinic. This suggestion is based on rare reports of significant, even fatal hemoperitoneum after liver aspiration. This rare event can even occur in the absence of coagulation defects.[8] (This report does not mention the size of the needle used for liver aspiration. We emphasize use of the smallest possible instrument.)

## Case 7

### Clinical History

Five years earlier, this 82-year-old woman had undergone a left modified radical mastectomy for infiltrating ductal carcinoma with axillary lymph node metastases. She was undergoing rheumatologic evaluation for joint pain when a 2 cm, firm, left anterior cervical lymph node was discovered. This mass was felt clinically to be most consistent with metastatic carcinoma. Its firm texture and recent appearance lent credence to this impression. Other possibilities included a wide range of reactive, neoplastic, and infectious causes of lymphadenopathy. Diagnosis required tissue sampling by either FNA or surgical excision.

### Fine-Needle Aspiration

No specialized techniques were required. Two aspirations with 25-gauge (0.5 mm) needles yielded gray, semisolid material sufficient for preparing 10 smears. Five were dried, and five were spray-fixed.

### Cytologic Findings

Eight smears showed only necrosis, with finely granular material. Although giant cells were not encountered, this material was identical to the background granularity seen in Figure 2.14. Two smears showed small granulomatous tissue fragments similar to those in Figure 2.15. (These were also set in a background of necrotic debris.)

Necrotizing, granulomatous lymphadenitis was diagnosed. This descriptive evaluation strongly suggested an infection with either mycobacterial or fungal agents. It did not completely exclude metastatic carcinoma as a diagnostic possibility because both necrosis and a granulomatous reaction may be associated with such lesions.

The cytologic picture in this case was typical of that seen in tuberculosis. No clinical imperative sufficient to warrant immediate surgery was operative. A repeat FNA was performed, and the material obtained was expressed into sterile saline and submitted to the laboratory of mycobacteriology and mycology, for culture of acid-fast and fungal organisms. As is frequently the case in immunocompetent individuals, the organism burden was too low to give positive results when special stains for organisms were applied to centrifuged fluid. Using radiometric technology, mycobacteria were identified in 10 days. These were later shown to represent *Mycobacterium tuberculosis*. Appropriate therapy was instituted without the need for surgery.

### Clinical Impact of FNA

Most of the cases we have heretofore considered involved diagnosis, classification, and staging of malignancies. This case presents a patient thought to harbor recurrence of a previously diagnosed carcinoma. The unexpected finding of a treatable infection is always welcome in this setting. One is occasionally in the unpleasant position of diagnosing a second malignancy.

Other general comments on culture of aspirated material are offered in Chapter 2 and summarized in Table 2.8.

## Case 8

### Clinical History

This 60-year-old male had chronic, severe cardiac and respiratory difficulties that made him a very poor surgical candidate. He was noted to have a 2-cm, soft parotid mass.

Evaluation by FNA was motivated by four factors: (1) This patient would be ill-advised to consider surgery under any but the most compelling circumstances; (2) most parotid masses are benign and can be safely left in place in this clinical setting; (3) parotid masses can be safely aspirated without danger of needle tract seeding, tumor dissemination, or damage to the facial nerve; (4) although uncommon tumors in this site may be very difficult to diagnose, the frequently encountered types of parotid neoplasms and inflammation are readily recognized in FNA material. These and other issues related to the diagnosis of parotid masses by FNA were discussed more fully in Chapter 2.

### Fine-Needle Aspiration

Using a 25-gauge (0.5 mm) needle, 0.5 cc of dark fluid was removed. Minimal size change occurred, so repeat FNA was performed, with similar results. These specimens were pooled and centrifuged. Smears were prepared from the pellet.

### Cytologic Findings

The fluid showed a background of proteinaceous precipitate and contained occasional crystals similar to those sometimes seen in thyroid-cyst fluids (see Color Plate XIII). Numerous free-lying lymphocytes made up the background cellular elements. Scattered through the smears were several large, cohesive sheets of epithelial cells. These showed the round nuclei, small nucleoli, and abundant finely granular cytoplasm of oncocytes (Figure 3.14). One fragment showed lymphoid tissue capped by tall, columnar oncocytes (Figure 3.15).

Figure 3.14.
*The smear from a Warthin's tumor of the parotid gland contained large sheets of oncocytic cells with round nuclei and abundant, granular cytoplasm (Papanicolaou stain, ×400 before a 34% reduction).*

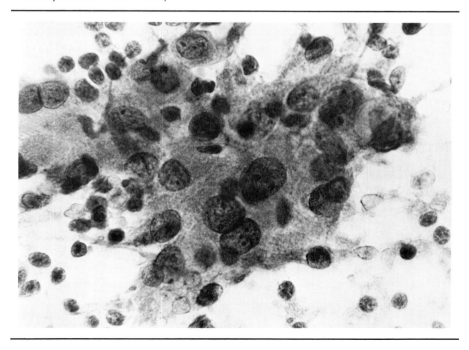

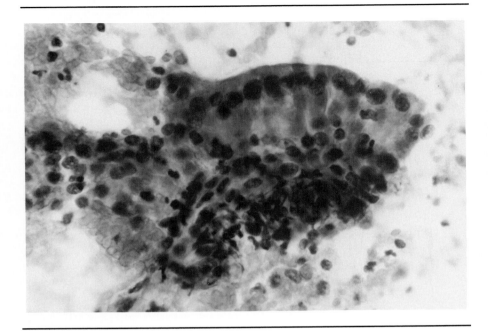

Figure 3.15.
*This tissue fragment shows small, darkly staining lymphocytes capped by tall, columnar oncocytes (Papanicolaou stain, ×400 before a 28% reduction).*

These features make up the typical cytologic presentation of Warthin's tumor (papillary cystadenoma lymphomatosum). The cell group shown in Figure 3.15 recapitulates the histopathology of this neoplasm quite well.

### Clinical Impact of FNA

Firm cytologic diagnosis of a specific benign neoplasm meant that surgery could be avoided in this high-risk patient.

## Case 9

### Clinical History

This 24-year-old female was referred for evaluation of a 2-cm firm thyroid nodule. The remaining areas of the gland were normal to palpation. Thyroid-function studies had not yet been evaluated.

Masses and generalized enlargements of the thyroid are very common. Many of these represent dominant nodules in multinodular goiter (nodular hyperplasia). Thyroid malignancy, on the other hand, is uncommon. Factors that might increase one's suspicion of malignancy include the finding of a single nodule, a male patient, age greater than 40 years, and a very firm lesion. In most instances, aspiration will be performed early in the patient's evaluation and only the information obtained by physical examination will be available. Thus, this 24-

year-old woman with a single firm nodule was clinically suspected to suffer from a thyroid malignancy.

### Fine-Needle Aspiration

Methods for safe and accurate aspiration of the thyroid were discussed in Chapter 2. This firm, 2-cm mass represented a technically straightforward problem. The aspirated material showed small amounts of blood, containing numerous grossly visible tissue particles. These smeared easily, indicating that they did not represent inadvertently recovered skeletal muscle (see **Case 5**).

### Cytologic Findings

Two distinct components were present. The first was polymorphous, benign-appearing lymphoid tissue featuring lymphocytes of various sizes, occasional plasma cells, and histiocytes. This component was similar to that depicted in Figure 2.13. In striking contrast were numerous cohesive groups of large cells (Figure 3.16). These showed large nuclei, occasional nucleoli, and moderate amounts of granular cytoplasm. A diagnosis of chronic lymphocytic (Hashimoto's) thyroiditis was rendered.

Figure 3.16.
*This case of chronic lymphocytic (Hashimoto's) thyroiditis showed numerous benign lymphoid cells similar to those in Figure 2.13. Groups such as the one shown here were also numerous. These large cells with abundant granular cytoplasm and somewhat pleomorphic nuclei represent the Hürthle cell component of this lesion (modified Diff-Quik® stain, ×500 before a 34% reduction).*

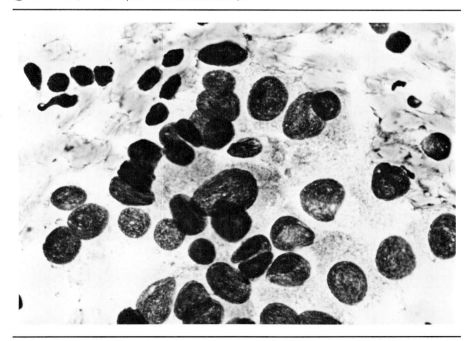

*Clinical Impact of FNA*

The typical patient with chronic lymphocytic thyroiditis (Hashimoto's disease) is generally said to be hypothyroid, with mild to moderate, diffuse, symmetrical thyromegaly. In our experience, clinical findings at presentation of autoimmune thyroiditis are actually quite variable. Patients who are hypothyroid often have a small or nonpalpable (presumably atrophic) gland. We have seen several individuals with this disorder who were clinically euthyroid and presented with a solitary nodule in an otherwise palpably normal gland. These patients are often referred for FNA by clinicians who suspect carcinoma. The diagnosis of thyroiditis is a welcome surprise.

When needed, confirmation of this diagnosis can be obtained in two ways: (1) Even in patients with early disease, there should be increased levels of thyroid stimulating hormone (TSH) in a majority of instances; levels may be abnormal before there is chemical or clinical evidence of hypothyroidism. (2) Even when the physical examination shows a solitary nodule, other areas of the gland are often involved by the inflammatory process. Finding changes similar to those we have illustrated in other areas of the gland supports the diagnosis of a diffuse condition. One can aspirate the opposite thyroid lobe by directing the needle to its normal location (see Figures 2.2 and 2.3). Even in the absence of palpable abnormalities, inflammation and Hürthle cell metaplasia indicative of thyroiditis can often be detected.

# Case 10

This discussion centers around an issue rather than a single patient. Aspirations that are not clinically helpful occur from time to time in virtually all body sites. These may be false negatives in which a malignancy is either not sampled or not appreciated. Alternatively, tissue may be obtained but may not adequately explain the clinical findings. We have chosen lymph-node FNA to illustrate some of these problems.

Lymphoid tissue (benign or malignant) can often be recovered in relatively pure form, with minimal blood. This material appears as small, gray, mucoid droplets when expressed from the needle. When spread and dried, it has a ground-glass appearance that we find helpful in being sure that appropriate tissue has been obtained (Figure 3.17). If appreciable blood is present, the tissue can often be seen as small, gray, glistening particles. These will spread out as the smear is prepared. In this setting, small areas of the blood film may be interrupted by islands showing the ground-glass appearance, as illustrated in Figure 3.17.

When clinical evidence of adenopathy is strong, and smears show only fat, blood, or nonspreading fragments suggestive of skeletal muscle (see Case 5), it should be assumed that the lesion has not been well sampled, and FNA should be repeated. In the cases discussed subsequently, however, histopathologic explanations for some grossly and cytologically nondiagnostic lymph-node aspirations are illustrated.

It is very important that such studies be regarded as nondiagnostic (that is, nonhelpful) rather than taken as evidence against a possible malignancy. Clinical findings that are not explained by the cytologic diagnosis should compel the

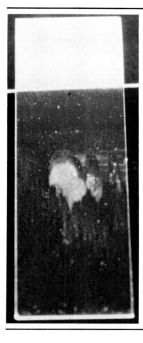

Figure 3.17.
*Pure lymphoid tissue with minimal blood has been spread and dried. It shows a translucent, gray, granular surface, similar to the ground glass that forms the slide's label. The white color of this smear indicates the nearly bloodless nature of this highly cellular preparation.*

physician to further investigation. This may include repeat FNA, surgical excision, or aspiration of an alternative site if multifocal disease is present.

### Densely Fibrous Malignant Neoplasms

Many malignancies elicit an inflammatory response from the host. The nature and extent of this reaction varies widely, but two neoplasms that are frequently sclerotic are breast carcinoma and Hodgkin's disease. Other adenocarcinomas and non-Hodgkin's lymphomas may also show sclerosis. Indeed, it is fibrosis that often accounts for the extremely firm texture of these lesions when the patient is examined or when the mass is penetrated by an aspiration needle.

In some cases, most of the pathologic tissue volume is composed of fibrous tissue. Such a case of Hodgkin's disease is illustrated in Figure 3.18. Only the very small, darkly stained foci contain cellular neoplastic tissue. Very thorough sampling is needed if such masses are to yield diagnostic material when aspirated.

Another fibrous lesion is the small breast carcinoma discussed in **Case 2** (see Figure 3.5). Aspiration yielded diagnostic cells (see Figure 3.4), albeit in very low numbers.

The clinical findings associated with masses such as that seen in Figure 3.18, or the radiographic manifestations of the small breast carcinoma in Figure 3.5 indicate that negative FNA results leave the clinical problem unresolved (see Table 2.2). It is imperative that diagnosis by other means be initiated.

When the entire FNA process outlined in Table 2.3 is carried out by a single individual, recognition of inadequate evaluation by FNA and recommendation of appropriate action will occur. Similarly, when a cytopathologist evaluates

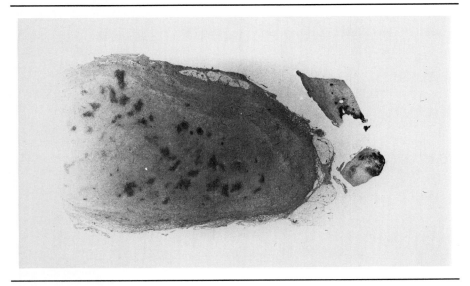

Figure 3.18.
*This whole-mount section shows a lymph node involved by nodular sclerosing Hodgkin's disease. The light areas are composed of hypocellular collagenous tissue. Only the small, darkly staining foci represent cellular areas of neoplastic tissue (H&E, whole-mount histologic section).*

material aspirated by a surgeon, oncologist, or other physician with experience in diagnosis and management of these lesions, appropriate actions will usually follow the nondiagnostic FNA.

Other physicians who are less experienced with oncologic problems may mistakenly interpret a nondiagnostic FNA report as definitely excluding malignancy as a diagnostic possibility. These individuals may not be fully aware that FNA has a small false-negative rate. The probability of error increases if the cytopathologist somewhat misleadingly indicates that the specimen is "negative for malignancy" rather than "nondiagnostic" or "inadequate." This danger is heightened when the individual performing the microscopy has not been made aware that the physical or radiographic findings strongly suggest malignancy. If the provocative nature of the physical findings have not been appreciated by a busy referring clinician (whose expertise may lie in other areas), the danger of error is very great.

We take this final opportunity to emphasize the value of the clinician–cytopathologist hybrid who both performs the aspiration and performs the microscopy. Given adequate training and experience, such physicians will skillfully perform the physical examination, obtain the best possible sample, provide optimum specimen preparation, and interpret the cytologic findings with circumspection. Either accurate diagnosis or recognition that FNA is noncontributory will result. Detailed communication among the several physicians caring for the patient is essential.

### Extensive Fatty Replacement of Lymph Nodes

Some lymph nodes show extensive fatty replacement. They will retain a delicate fibrous capsule associated with a thin rim of lymphoid tissue. Except for this peripheral band (often microscopic in width), the node is entirely replaced by adipose tissue (Figure 3.19). Our experience dissecting surgical specimens indicates that this phenomenon is quite common in lymph nodes of the axilla.

The fibrous capsule renders these nodes easily palpable, both in vivo and in surgical specimens. Thus, they are occasionally selected as targets for FNA. Fatty replacement can be suspected when smears show adipose tissue and small amounts of lymphoid tissue. Given the technical difficulties that attend FNA of small axillary masses, one generally suspects that the lesion has been poorly sampled or missed altogether. (In the neck, missing a lymph node usually yields smears containing skeletal muscle. In other sites, adipose tissue will usually be recovered.)

Repeat FNA may yield more diagnostic tissue. The technique illustrated in Figure 2.9 can help ensure that the needle is accurately placed within the palpable mass. In some cases, only surgical excision will provide sufficient diagnostic certainty.

### Apparent Lymph Nodes That Are Not Lymph Nodes

We are occasionally asked to aspirate apparent lesions that are normal structures. This is most common when thin individuals seem to have palpable abnormalities in the neck. Bones of the cervical spine, laryngeal cartilages,

Figure 3.19.
*This lymph node shows a thin rim of lymphoid tissue and a delicate capsule. It is otherwise replaced by adipose tissue (H&E, whole-mount histologic section).*

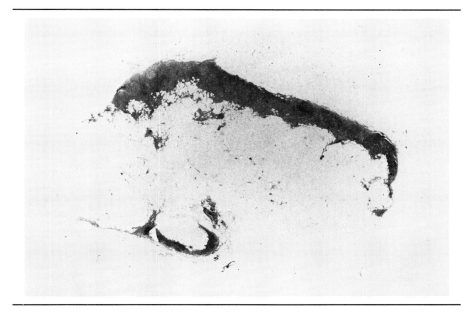

portions of the carotid system and even tendinous structures have all been referred for FNA. Careful physical examination can solve some of these problems, especially when symmetrical, contralateral palpatory findings can be identified.

Bones of the cervical spine are sometimes mistaken for deep-seated adenopathy. Asymmetry may heighten this suspicion and may be associated with pain and changes of degenerative joint disease. The nature of these masses is immediately apparent when the aspirating needle contacts bone. Smears will have variable combinations of blood, adipose tissue, and skeletal muscle. Radiographic studies may confirm the skeletal nature of some such pseudo lymph nodes.[9]

Breast tissue can be present in the midline over the sternum, as high as the clavicles, and in the axilla. Benign and malignant conditions can involve this tissue. This poses a clinical problem when enlarged breast tissue in the axilla is clinically believed to represent pathologic adenopathy. FNA will yield variable amounts of adipose tissue and breast epithelial cells. If thorough sampling is achieved, the identification of benign breast tissue will suffice to explain the clinical findings. One example of such axillary breast tissue that was clinically suspected to represent pathologic lymphadenopathy is shown in Figure 3.20.

### Extensively Necrotic Lymph Nodes

Lymph-node infarction is uncommon but may be associated with vasculitis, infectious lymphadenitis, trauma, or malignant lymphoma.[10] Infarction as an apparent consequence of FNA is exceedingly rare.[11] Necrotic material that may be completely devoid of viable cells can be aspirated from lymph nodes replaced

Figure 3.20.
*This breast tissue presented in the axilla and was clinically felt to represent lymphadenopathy. Most of this mass is fatty. The thin fibrous septa—seen as dark lines in this preparation—contain small, normal-appearing breast ducts (H&E, whole-mount histologic section).*

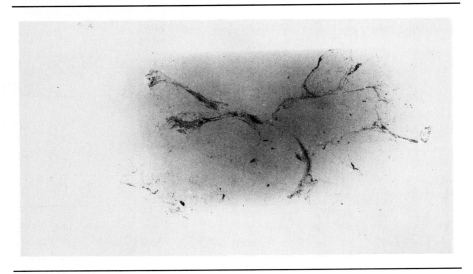

by infectious or malignant processes. We have noted this most often when aspirating tuberculous nodes. FNA may yield abundant semisolid or fluid material that may contain small particles.

Once necrotic material has been carefully examined for granulomas, identifiable organisms, or tumor cells, repeat FNA can provide additional material for both culture and further microscopic study. If malignant cells are not identified, diagnosis must await culture results. A more detailed consideration of culture in FNA can be found in Chapter 2 (see Table 2.8).

# REFERENCES

1. Zajicek J: Aspiration biopsy cytology: Part I. Cytology of supradiaphragmatic organs, pp. 171–179. Basel, Karger, Switzerland:1974.
2. Silverman JF, Lannin DR, O'Brien K, Norris HT: The triage role of fine needle aspiration of palpable breast masses: Diagnostic accuracy and cost-effectiveness. Acta Cytol 1987;31:731–736.
3. Frable WJ: Letter to the editor. Hum Pathol 1989;20:1133.
4. Stanley MW, Tani EM, Rutquist LE, Skoog L: Cystosarcoma phyllodes of the breast: A cytologic and clinicopathologic study of 23 cases. Diagn Cytopathol 1989; 5:29–34.
5. Johnston WW, Frable WJ: Diagnostic respiratory cytopathology, pp. 224–235. Masson Publishing, 1979.
6. Rosenthal DL: Cytopathology of pulmonary disease, pp. 140–141. Basel, Switzerland: Karger, 1988.
7. Olynyk PW, Williams P, Fudge A, et al.: Fine-needle aspiration biopsy for the measurement of hepatic iron concentration. Hepatology 1991;15:502–506.
8. Edoute Y, Kaplan J, Ben-Haim SA, Baruch Y: Hæmoperitoneum induced by fine needle aspiration of liver in patients with disseminated intravascular coagulation. Lancet 1992; 339: 121–122.
9. Stanley MW, Knoedler J: Skeletal pseudo-lymph nodes of the neck: A clinical problem addressed by fine needle aspiration. Diagn Cytopathol: In Press.
10. Cleary KR, Osborne BM, Butler JJ: Lymph node infarction foreshadowing malignant lymphoma. Am J Surg Pathol 1982;6:435–442.
11. Dekmezian RH, Sneige N, Katz RL: The effect of fine needle aspiration on lymph node morphology in lymphoproliferative disorders. Acta Cytol 1989;33:732–733.

# Index

Note: Page numbers in italics refer to figures; page numbers followed by t refer to tables.